Issues in Heart Failure Nursing

Forthcoming titles from M&K Publishing

Self Assessment in –
Limb X-ray Interpretation
ISBN 978 1-905539-13-4

Improving Patient Outcomes: a guide for Ward Managers
ISBN 978 -1-905539-06-1

Modern Management in Chronic Disease & Long Term Conditions
ISBN 978-1-905539-15-4

The ECG Workbook
ISBN 978-1-905539-14-7

Emergency Management for Nurses
ISBN 978 1-905539-05-3

Nurse Facilitated Hospital Discharge
ISBN 978 -1-905539-12-6

The Advanced Respiratory Practitioner:
a practical & theoretical guide for Nurses & AHPs
ISBN 978-1-905539-10-9

Pre-Operative Assessment and Perioperative Management
ISBN 978 1-905539-02-9

Pre-teen and Teenage Pregnancy: a 21st century reality
ISBN 978 1-905539-11-8

Nurse Consultancy
ISBN 978-1-905539-09-3

Eye Emergencies: The practitioner's guide
ISBN 978 1-905539-08-6

Managing Emotions in Women's Health
ISBN 978 1-905539-07-X

Issues in Heart Failure Nursing

Edited by

Chris Jones
Senior Lecturer, Faculty Of Health
Edge Hill University, Aintree Hospital Campus

Foreword by

Professor Martin Cowie
Professor of Cardiology (Health Services Research),
Imperial College London
Honorary Consultant, Royal Brompton Hospital

M&K Publishing
©2006 M&K Update Ltd.

First published 2006

Notice:
Clinical practice and medical knowledge constantly evolve. Standard safety precautions must be followed, but as knowledge is broadened by research, changes in practice, treatment and drug therapy may become necessary or appropriate. Readers must check the most current product information provided by the manufacturer of each drug to be administered and verify the dosages and correct administration, as well as contraindications. It is the responsibility of the practitioner, utilising the experience and knowledge of the patient, to determine dosages and the best treatment for each individual patient. Neither the publisher nor the authors assume any liability for any injury and/or damage to persons or property arising from this publication.

The Publisher

To contact M&K Publishing write to:
M&K Update Ltd · The Old Bakery · St. John's Street · Keswick · Cumbria · CA12 5AS
a part of M&K Update Ltd

Tel: 01768 773030 · Fax: 01768 781099
publishing@mkupdate.co.uk
www.mkupdate.co.uk

British Library Catalogue in Publication Data
A catalogue record for this book is available from the British Library

ISBN: 978-1-905539-00-0

Designed by Mary Blood
Typeset in 11pt Usherwood Book
Printed in United Kingdom by Reed's Ltd., Penrith.

Contents

List of contributors

Contributors

Debbie Bell RN, Dip CHD/Heart Failure
Lead Practice Nurse/QOF Lead, Family Surgery, Southport

Marj Carey Dip He, RN
Community Heart Failure Specialist Nurse
Knowsley Primary Care Trust

Sarah Ellison RN, BSc(Hons)
Heart Failure Specialist Nurse, Cheshire West Primary Care Trust

Barbara Flowers BSc, RN
Cardiac Support Nurse, Southport and Ormskirk NHS Trust

Robert Frodsham RN, BSc
Charge Nurse, Coronary Care Unit,
St Helens and Knowsley NHS Trust, Merseyside

Christine Gardner RN
Cardiac Advisory Nurse/Heart Failure Lead, Central Liverpool
Primary Care Trust and Clinical Lead Nurse with the
Cheshire and Merseyside Cardiac Network

Linda Gladman RN
Staff Nurse, Coronary Care Unit, Whiston Hospital, Merseyside

Chris Jones MSc, BA, RN, RNT, PGCE, ENB 100
Senior Lecturer, Faculty of Health, Edge Hill University,
University Hospital Aintree, Liverpool

Michelle Kerr
Sister, Cardiac Rehabilitation Service,
University Hospital Aintree, Liverpool

Joanne Lackey RN, BA (Hons), Dip HE
Senior Sister, Coronary Care Unit,
University Hospital Aintree, Liverpool

Clare Lewis RGN, BSc (Hons)
Community Matron, South Sefton Primary Care Trust, Merseyside

Barbara Stephens MSc, BA (Hons), DPSN, RGN
Nurse Consultant for Heart Failure Management,
University Hospital Aintree, Liverpool

Pippa Witter RGN, DN, CPT, BSc (Hons), BA (Hons)
Community Matron, Southport and formby Primary Care Trust

Foreword

As the number of people with heart failure rises year-on-year, and the range of treatment options that can be considered increases, the challenge is for the patient not to become 'lost' in the process of delivering high-quality multidisciplinary care. The nurse has a key role to play in ensuring a holistic approach is adopted. This book has been written by those with much practical experience of working with people living, and dying, with heart failure.

Many questions will be raised by patients and their families, and not just about the diagnosis and possible treatments. How can the symptoms be controlled? What about exercise? Is sexual activity still possible? What will happen at 'the end'? In this book, such topics are covered from a practical viewpoint, by those who deal with these issues every day. Unlike many texts, difficult issues are neither ignored nor glossed over.

People with heart failure often have other health problems that complicate the advice that should be given on treatment and monitoring. Those with cognitive dysfunction and other mental health problems are particularly poorly served at present. This book raises some of the key issues that may need to be considered. It also addresses the increasing number of people who have been living with heart problems since birth who then develop heart failure. Such patients are often expert in managing their condition, and their information needs may be quite different from those who have never before had a heart problem.

Despite the best efforts of the entire health care team, life expectancy is inevitably reduced for patients with heart failure. Recent advances in the assessment of palliative care needs, and the best way of addressing these, are discussed at some length and will be a great help to health care professionals.

No one who reads this book will be left in any doubt that while much is improving, much remains to be tackled. Guidelines are the backbone of modern clinical practice, but they can only inform practice. Political efforts, such as the National Service Framework and the Quality and Outcomes Framework of the new General Medical Services contract for primary care, direct clinical efforts in certain – albeit limited – directions.

Foreword

Important and valuable as these initiatives may be, many crucial aspects of the holistic approach to care for a person living with heart failure are not specifically mentioned or rewarded. This should not discourage us in our efforts to deliver the highest possible standard of care.

As the NHS is constantly being redesigned, many professional roles are changing. This book encourages readers to challenge their preconceptions and to think about the skills that different professionals have, and how they might be harnessed for the benefit of patients.

Heart failure is a challenge for everyone. This book is a welcome addition to the literature, and brings together some of the topics often not discussed at professional meetings or in larger texts.

Difficult questions remain, not least about how to ensure everyone with heart failure in the UK gains access to high quality and responsive care. However, all nurses caring for patients with heart failure will be enriched by sharing the experiences of those who have contributed to this book.

Martin R Cowie
Professor of Cardiology, Imperial College
and Honorary Consultant Cardiologist,
Royal Brompton Hospital, London.

Preface

In March 2005 a feature article in *The Observer Magazine* raised the subject of the oncoming crisis of chronic illness and, in particular, the oncoming crisis due to heart failure. Crisis is hardly too strong a word. The number of people suffering from this debilitating condition is predicted to grow exponentially over the next decade. This has serious implications for the health services. Investigating heart failure is not cheap even where facilities exist. Echocardiographers are highly trained professionals who require a lot of preparatory training. Treating patients is not cheap. The drugs used, though effective – often remarkably so – are also costly and mandate laboratory investigations. These again are not cheap. People with heart failure require frequent admissions to hospital and occupy many beds and much staff attention. All of these factors are set to increase over the next decades.

Paradoxically the growth in the numbers of people suffering from heart failure reflects improvements in the treatment of people with ischaemic heart disease and hypertension. People now survive heart attacks because their coronary arteries are opened up promptly following infarct. This may well preserve their lives, but it also allows them to survive with a damaged, compromised heart that may quickly show signs of insufficiency. Although they may respond well to treatment, the overall prospects for these patients are still bleak.

Public policy developments have begun to take the problem of heart failure seriously. Landmarks included the National Service Framework for heart disease, which started the ball rolling by having a chapter devoted to the subject of heart failure. Following this the National Institute for Clinical Excellence issued guidelines. These were welcome developments and outlined the 'industry standard' level of treatment a patient could expect, regardless of postcode. The problem was that these developments led to an increase in the demand placed on already stretched services. New thinking was called for and new approaches to old problems demanded.

One of these new approaches was the development of nurse-led services to manage the day-to-day progress of patients. Both in hospital and in the community these services have proved

Preface

more than effective in meeting this growing demand, and have managed to reduce the requirement for emergency admissions to hospital. Having a friendly and familiar nurse to give advice and help with day-to-day difficulties can make all the difference to an elderly person who is struggling to manage complex medication regimes.

Of course the nurses who are taking up the role of caring for patients with heart failure have their own needs and requirements. Foremost among these needs is enhanced education and training. Heart failure has many complex and difficult aspects to consider of a technical and an interpersonal nature. Yet heart failure nurses had precious little educational opportunities for educational support in their new roles. Specifically designed higher education modules have been few and far between. The British Heart Foundation has supported some excellent initiatives in London and in Glasgow, but the rest of the country has been poorly served.

It was to meet this need that one of the contributors to this book, Barbara Stephens, suggested that Edge Hill University develop a course in heart failure for people who were involved in the care of this group of patients. The take up of places on the module has proven Barbara's initial hunch to be correct. The participants in this module have been nurses whose experience in the field has been vast, but whose academic recognition has been low. Our module 'Meeting the Challenge of Heart Failure' has permitted these nurses to demonstrate their mastery of this demanding area.

Though the module is still relatively new and at the time of writing has run eight times, it has generated nine articles which have been accepted for publication. These have focused on many different aspects of the care of these patients, but in the main have highlighted challenges and dilemmas faced by nurses and the patients they care for. It is these pieces of work which form the basis of this book. Reviewed, revised and brought up to date for another audience, this collection of essays addresses a wide range of topics. The previously published material is referenced where appropriate.

It is a tribute to the seniority and the skill of these course participants that so many of their assignments were accepted for publication. Yet I am convinced that many, many more could have done so had they submitted their work for consideration. Nevertheless this collection represents the views and the ideas of staff dealing with the problems of heart failure in hospital and in the community. These are the people who will be in the front line in meeting the challenge of heart failure.

The book is intended for people caring for patients with heart failure and addresses issues and dilemmas in the care of this client group. As such the book assumes a certain amount of understanding of the pathophysiology and the treatment of this distressing condition.

Chris Jones
Senior Lecturer, Faculty of Health
Edge Hill University, St Helens Road, Ormskirk, Lancashire

Editor's note

Editor's note

Throughout the text reference will be made to the New York Heart Association classification of heart failure symptoms. For reference purposes the classifications are listed in the appendix on page 152.

Chapter 1

Heart Failure in the Community
A confusion of protocols? [1]

Debbie Bell

Introduction

If it was ever possible for community nurses to practice in a way
which was not supported by research-based theory, those days
are long gone. In the modern era, evidence-based protocols are
issued in profusion to guide and mandate practice. This chapter
aims to examine the standards and clinical protocols that are
currently utilised in general practice, for the management of
heart failure patients.

Accordingly, this chapter will compare and contrast those
chapters of the National Service Framework (NSF) for Coronary
Heart Disease which deal with heart failure, (DoH 2000a) the
National Institute for Clinical Excellence (NICE) guidelines
relating to heart failure and the General Medical Services (GMS)
contractual obligations relating to heart failure. All of these have
different things to offer the heart failure patient.

Background

In July 2000 the government published 'The NHS Plan: A plan for
investment a plan for reform' (DoH 2000b). In its preface it
recognised the failings of the National Health Service (NHS) in
keeping up with changes in our society. A major investment was
to be initiated in the NHS, to modernise and reform it.

One of the key intentions of this investment was to 'reshape
the NHS from a patient's point of view' (p.3). Ten key principles

of service were put forward which included features such as: health promotion, disease prevention, cultural needs and improving quality services. This is not an exhaustive list. The advent of the NSF for coronary heart disease (CHD) in 2000 which included a chapter targeted solely at heart failure, aimed to provide a cohesive approach to diagnosis, treatment, continuing care and health promotion for heart failure patients.

In 2003 the National Institute for Clinical Excellence (NICE) then produced its guidelines for patients with heart failure. These, according to Mayor (2003) were 'designed to clarify the best practice for health professionals caring for adult patients, who have or who are suspected of having heart failure'. Then, when the NICE and the NSF guidelines were shaping the medical treatment offered to patients a different voice was heard. This was in the shape of the General Medical Council-backed General Medical Services contract for GPs, which was in place from April 2003 (NHS Confederation).

The intention of this contract was to pay doctors for services rendered and to reward quality performance by linking payment to the attainment of quality indicators, in this case to those which pertain to patients with heart failure. Currently three indicators relate to the care of patients with failing cardiac performance or left ventricular dysfunction (LVD): first, that practices produce a register for heart failure patients; second, that their diagnosis is confirmed by ECG or by echocardiogram; third, that patients deemed to have LVD should be prescribed an Angiotensin Converting Enzyme (ACE) inhibitor or an angiotensin receptor antagonist.

Immediately, a problem becomes apparent which sits at the heart of all these initiatives. There is no mention in the GMS quality indicators of treating these patients with diuretics, digoxin, warfarin or spironolactone. And yet these same substances are mentioned in both the NICE and the NSF documents. So either the GMS quality indicators are missing out important therapies, or the NSF and NICE guidelines are including therapies which can be regarded as optional extras to quality care.

In order to examine whether there are other inconsistencies between these guidelines, I intend to examine the case of an entirely fictitious patient John, who has been diagnosed as having 'a complex syndrome that can result from any structural or functional cardiac disorder, that impairs the ability of the heart to function as a pump to support a physiological circulation' (NICE 2003). In other words heart failure.

Case history

Case history

John is a 54-year-old bricklayer, married with two children, he is an ex-smoker and drinks a minimal amount of alcohol. His body mass index (BMI) is 27, and his most recent blood pressure (B/P) was 136/74. Both his mother and father had angina; in addition his father suffered a myocardial infarction at the age of 60. Both parents are still living. He has asthma, which is well controlled.

In July 2000 he consulted his general practitioner because of an increasing dyspnoea and cough. His chest X-ray revealed 'nothing of note' with the lungs normal and the heart size normal. To be on the safe side his GP requested an echo. Events overtook the patient however when increasing angina type central, crushing and radiating chest pain took John to hospital. He revealed on this occasion that he had been experiencing an increase in breathlessness at work, difficulties sleeping flat and 'palpitations'. His blood pressure was found to be low. An echo was performed immediately which revealed a dilated left ventricle whose walls were moving poorly. This was also the case with his right ventricle. As if this was not bad enough, the dilation of the ventricle had resulted in a 'moderate to severe' mitral regurgitation. After treatment and stabilisation John was sent back home. His medication consisted of digoxin, warfarin, frusemide, spironolactone, losartan and glyceril trinitrate (GTN).

The discharge letter from the hospital indicated that John had developed an idiopathic dilated cardiomyopathy which resulted in both ventricles failing. Arrangements were put in place for him to see his cardiologist in twelve weeks. Routine primary care monitoring brought him to the attention of the district nursing service.

When he attended surgery he had his liver and thyroid function tested, his fasting levels of glucose and cholesterol were measured and a full blood count was performed. The only problem area was a mildly elevated cholesterol level, which was treated with lipid lowering agents and advice from the dietician.

In addition he was invited to attend the practice to have his asthma checked and was also given an annual review date to assess his status as a patient with established heart disease. This extra attention was not because he was getting worse. On the contrary, he reported that his condition was stable. He understood his condition well and co-operated in his treatment even to the extent of joining a gym for weight reducing exercise.

Comparison of protocols

Comparison of protocols

The details of this somewhat typical case of a person with heart failure are designed to bring out some interesting differences between the NSF and NICE guidelines and those of the GMS contract.

The NSF for heart failure allows for the provision of key investigations to aid diagnosis. These include a 12 lead ECG, echo and also suggest chest X-ray, renal function tests, weight, and haemoglobin measurement. Before his admission to hospital, John had undergone a chest X-ray and was waiting for an echo. Had he presented today (2005) with these same symptoms, then the 2003 NICE guidelines would recommend the same initial investigations, but with the addition of an assay for the presence in blood of abnormal amounts of Brain Natriuretic Peptides (BNP). While numerous conditions can elevate levels of BNP, normal levels may exclude a diagnosis of heart failure.

If basic investigations do not indicate heart failure then it further recommends an echo should be performed. This consolidates the diagnosis and more importantly gives a fuller picture on underlying functional abnormality of the heart. The GMS contract makes no provision for BNP tests to be performed.

Within some local Primary Care Trusts, there is at present no opportunity to perform routine BNP tests, which might exclude heart failure. This inevitably puts extra pressure on overworked echo services examining patients, many of whom may not have heart failure in the first place. Mead (2003) points out this is likely to become a serious problem as in many areas there are already lengthy waiting lists for an echo. It has been suggested by some observers that the extra money GPs will receive through the GMS contract could be used to purchase a hand-held echocardiograph machine. These machines are very expensive and could be shared between practices. Doctors who have an interest in cardiology may wish to offer this service to their patients. It would as suggested by Xiao (2003) allow GPs to offer point-of-care echocardiograms to patients suspected of having heart failure. He warns, however, that the doctor should undertake an intensive period of training as their interpretation requires more than a little experience and training.

Continuing care

Both the NSF and NICE guidelines stress the importance of further investigations to evaluate any other possible aggravating factors for heart failure. This might be done by performing tests such as chest X-ray, thyroid function tests, liver function tests, fasting lipids and glucose, urinalysis and peak flow spirometry. Under the GMS contract however, it is not obligatory that the investigations outlined above are offered. It is true that some of this ground might be covered by the quality indicators for coronary heart disease. The problem is that they might not be interpreted as being of relevance for heart failure also.

The British Hypertension Society's (Williams *et al.* 2004) guidelines for the management of hypertension state that a blood pressure reading of 150/90 mmHg should attract treatment. However, patients with diabetes, renal impairment or established cardiovascular disease, should aim for a target BP of 130/80 mmHg.

John's latest BP was 136/94 mmHg and this mild hypertension was treated with Losartan. In this case his GP would be awarded points for his blood pressure being less than 150/90, and payment would be made in recognition of this standard. However, ideally his blood pressure would only be controlled in line with the BHS recommendations when it reaches 130/80. This 'points make prizes' approach to care has been noted by many authors who point out that chasing the hypertensive patient and lowering his blood pressure to 150/90 'will be financially rewarding' (Mead 2003) while going the extra mile for patients with more complex conditions may not.

A similar confusion of guidelines can be seen in relation to the control of serum cholesterol. Here the recommendations are that total cholesterol should be reduced from less than 5mmol/l to less than 4mmol/l. At present, the NSF does not make any recommendation in chapter six about target levels for cholesterol in cases of heart failure. It does, however, recommend target levels in the chapter on preventing heart disease. The NICE guidelines suggest that patients, who have a combination of heart failure and atherosclerotic vascular disease, should receive statins. The GMS contract recommends a target level of less than 5mmol/s for total cholesterol, but only in patients with pre-existing coronary disease. It is not one of the quality indicators for left ventricular dysfunction.

Annual reviews

Annual reviews

All three documents agree that patients with a diagnosis of LVD should have regular reviews. However, what should be assessed at this annual review differs somewhat between the NSF, NICE guidelines and GMS contract. The NSF includes the following aspects of ideal continuing care: control of blood pressure, weight management, immunisation, cardiac rehabilitation, long-term social support, alcohol/nutritional/smoking status, physical activity and palliative care needs. These factors are addressed by the NICE guidelines, which also state the importance of good communication skills, which are needed during interactions with patients and their families.

Not only here do the NICE guidelines broach the subject of the more human side of the patient's care. Anxiety and depression tend to be more common in patients with heart failure, than in the general population (NICE 2003). In raising this subject NICE guidelines have addressed a major issue not really covered by the NSF or GMS contract, and yet this is perhaps one area that may give the patient and his/her family the most distress. Apart from the clinical symptoms, such as increased dyspnoea/fatigue and pain, the emotional and psychological effect of a terminal disease such as heart failure, can be as profound as the disease itself. Depression has been shown to increase the admission rates to the hospital setting (Gibbs *et al.* 2002) and this, they claim, is as a result of mental health problems in heart failure patients being overlooked, which can in fact lead to significant psychological distress.

At no time does the GMS contract address this issue, either in the coronary heart disease quality indicators or the LVD subset. It does however have indicators for mental health, which focus on those patients who are already diagnosed as having severe long-term mental health problems. These are not currently linked with LVD.

Measuring and monitoring treatment

Measuring and monitoring treatment

Measuring the severity of symptoms is always fraught with difficulty and it is hard to imagine a one-size-fits-all measuring device for the accurate measurement of disease progress and remission. However the New York Heart Association scale is widely used to measure progress, relapse and severity in heart failure. Certainly it is used in both the NSF and NICE guidelines to guide recommendations. In the GMS contract it is invisible. Perhaps it is regarded as a 'common sense' tool to be used in assessment and does not require a specific recommendation. But perhaps not.

End of life care

End of life care

Much work has been done in the provision of palliative services to patients with various forms of cancer, but the provision of palliative care offered to patients suffering from cardiac failure is inadequate. It is only within the last few years that there has been a recognition that heart failure patients desperately need, and rightly deserve, the much-acclaimed models of care that cancer patients receive.

It is perhaps unthinkable in today's society, that a patient with terminal cancer would not be offered palliative care in one form or another. However, the following words from a patient who is in end stage heart failure, suggest that there is still a long way to go, in achieving and providing palliative care to all heart failure patients. 'I was sitting in a chair all night, I would be screaming for air, very, very frightening. I suppose it's like drowning really' Murray *et al.* (2002).

These are very distressing words coming from someone who it is felt must have been in severe physiological, emotional and psychological pain. This extract was taken from a study conducted by Murray *et al.* (2002). Their objective was to compare the illness trajectories, needs and service use of cancer patients, and of those who had advanced cardiac failure. In its conclusion it highlighted that cardiac patients received far less palliative care, health and social services, than those patients who had terminal cancer.

It could be argued that the NSF only pays lip service to palliative care in its guidelines. It asks only that health care professionals 'consider the potential benefit of providing palliative care services and palliation aids' (p. 6). It does not offer any real structure or advice on how these services should be provided. Echoing the more human orientation of its recommendations outlined above, NICE discusses end of life issues with more clarity and empathy, however by its own admission it does stress that although it includes such issues as palliative care in its guidelines, it does not consider them in detail.

The GMS contract does not discuss non-cancer palliative care for heart failure patients at all. As discussed earlier, money is paid to the GP for every quality indicator achieved. Priority is given to the diagnosis and treatment of LVD. These indicators can quite easily be met. Maintaining the continued care that is needed by both patients and their families, and encompassing their palliative needs are harder tasks and altogether more gruelling. No financial incentives here may lead to a form of care delivery which may well be of a much lower standard. In general practice the vast majority of GPs and allied health professionals may well intend to provide the best care possible for their patients. However, when discussing the new contract Lewis and Gillam (2002) argued that all incentive systems can encourage 'gaming', and this they argue may lead GPs to concentrate on those quality targets which are specified, to the detriment of others.

Conclusion

During this chapter it has been the intention to compare and contrast the NSF, NICE guidelines and the new GMS contract, and discuss how they deliver, maintain and manage the patient with established heart failure. The discussion has ranged from diagnosis through continuing care and finally, has raised end of life issues. The areas listed in this discussion are by no means exhaustive. Many of the points raised in this discussion have derived from my own observations in the field of primary care. Of course it should be pointed out that all three documents had different policy priorities which pushed them forward, and each was intended to perform a different role. But still, each acts in its own way as a guide to practice and might be expected to point in the same direction in each of the important fields outlined above.

While the NSF provided a good canvas to work from, it is now in need of updating and further review. The NICE clinical guidelines provided a strategy for best practice in the investigations, treatment and support that should be offered to heart failure patients, with greater emphasis being placed on the human element of a terminal illness, e.g. communication skills and palliative care interventions. Finally, the GMS contract, which was introduced to primary care in April 2003, is very limited in its approach to the quality of care that should be afforded heart failure patients. It has a long way to go before it encompasses all the standards that should be met for those individuals who have to face life with heart failure.

Note
1. An earlier treatment of this subject was published in December 2004 in *Primary Health Care*, 14 (10), 27–31, and permission to adapt this chapter has been granted by that publisher..

Debbie Bell

The General Medical Services have had some revisions made to the original 2003 contract. In February 2006 these revisions were introduced for implementation in April 2006. The original contract had LVD (left ventricular dysfunction) as part of the CHD clinical indicators. This has now changed, and has been renamed as HEART FAILURE. The clinical indicators still remain the same as the 2003 GMS Contract

HF1: The practice can produce a register of patients with heart failure

Initial diagnosis

HF2: The percentage of patients with a diagnosis of heart failure (diagnosed after 1 April 2006) which has been confirmed by an echocardiogram or by specialist assessment

Ongoing management

HF3: The percentage of patients with a current diagnosis of heart failure due to LVD who are currently treated with an ACE inhibitor or Angiotensin Receptor Blocker, who can tolerate therapy and for whom there is no contra-indication

References

Department of Health (DoH) (2000a) *National Service Framework for Coronary Heart Disease.* London: Department of Health.

Department of Health (2000b). *The NHS Plan: A plan for investment, a plan for reform.* London: The Stationery Office.

Gibbs, J.S.R., McCoy, A.S.M., Gibbs, L.M.E., Rogers, A.E., & Addington-Hall, J.M. (2002). Living with and dying from heart failure: the role of palliative care. *Heart,* **88** (Oct), 1136–40.

Lewis, R. & Gillam, S. (eds.) (2002). A fresh new contract for General Practitioners. *British Medical Journal,* **324** (May), 1048–9.

Mayor, S. (2003). NICE issues new guidelines for patients with heart failure. *British Medical Journal,* **327** (7408), 179-a.

Mead, M. (2003). Cardiology and the new GMS contract for GPs. *British Journal of Cardiology,* **10** (5), 329–31.

Murray, S.A., Boyd, K., Kendall, M., Worth, A., Benton, T.F. & Clansen, H. (2002). Dying of lung cancer or cardiac failure. Prospective qualitative interview study of patients and their carers in the community. *British Medical Journal,* **325** (October) 929.

National Institute for Clinical Excellence (2003). *Chronic Heart Failure. Management of Chronic Heart Failure in Adults in Primary and Secondary Care.* London: NICE.

The NHS Confederation (2003). *New GMS Contract: Investing in General Practice.* London: The NHS Confederation.

Williams, B., Pulter, N.R., Brown, M.J., Davis, M., McInnes, G.T., Potter, J.P., Sever, P.S. & Thom, S. McG. The British Hypertension Society (BHS) Guidelines, Working Party Guidelines for Management of Hypertension; Report of the Fourth Working Party of BHS (2004). BHS IV. *Journal of Hypertension 2004,***18** 139–85.

Xiao, H. (2003). Hand-held echocardiography for primary care. *British Journal of Cardiology,* **10** (3) 235–40.

Bibliography

Ashrafian, H. (ed.) (2004). Portable echocardiography. *British Medical Journal,* **327**, 1181–2.

Davies, P. & Glasspool, J. (eds.) (2003). Patients and the new contracts. *British Medical Journal,* **326**, 1099.

Flint, J. (ed.) (2003). The expert patient: good thinking or a cross-to bear? *British Journal of Cardiology.* **10**, 11–13.

Hobbs, F.D.R., Davies, R.C. & Lip, G.Y.H. (2000). ABC of heart failure in general practice. *British Medical Journal,* **320**, 626–9.

West, R. (2004). Assessment of dependence and motivation to stop smoking. *British Medical Journal,* **328**, 338–9.

Whyler, D. (2003). CHD: the provision of services to patients in primary care. *Cardiology News,* **6**, (6) 13–15.

Wilson, A., Pearson, D. & Hassey, A. (2002). *Barriers to developing the nurse practitioner role in primary care – the GP perspective. Family Practice,* **19**, (6) 641–6.

Vasan, R. (ed.) (2003). Diastolic heart failure. *British Medical Journal,* **327**, (Nov.), 1181–2.

Chapter 2

District nurses meeting the challenge of heart failure[1]

Pippa Witter

District nurses and patient empowerment

Patient empowerment

In recent years there has been a revolution in the approach of the health services in caring for patients. It has been nowhere more in evidence than in the care of people in their own homes. District nurses have been in the forefront of these developments.

The developments in public policy which have driven this transformation were first the NHS plan (2000) and second the Cancer plan (2000). Both these documents set out to transform the delivery of services in line with the demands of a new century and a population more versed in demanding services tailored to the needs of the clients using them. The watchwords became involvement, empowerment and top to bottom modernisation. Of course such a radical break, from an ethos which traditionally relied on the passive acceptance by patients of services aimed at them, called for wholesale rethinking by the health care professions. This was especially so in the areas of service organisation, quality assurance, recruitment, leadership, workforce planning and education (Bullen 2002). For a time it seemed that there was an endless stream of documents each signalling a more radical vision of the future of health care delivery, much of which had nursing as its direct focus. *Meeting the Challenge* (DoH 2000a), *Making a Difference* (DoH 1999), *The Nursing Contribution to Cancer Care* (DoH 2000c) all gave professionals food for thought in these debates, but if two themes were to be picked out which underpinned the discussion these could be said to be *partnership* and *leadership* (Bullen 2002).

Pippa Witter

The recommendations of this torrent of public policy initiatives have in large part fallen on district nurses to implement. This was acknowledged in the review of progress made by the Department of Health in 2003 entitled 'Maintaining the Momentum'. Reviewing the delivery of cancer services, the pivotal role of district nursing in the delivery of services was highlighted. The review went on to favourably comment on educational initiatives designed to enable patients diagnosed with cancer to live and die at home during their terminal phase. The Macmillan Gold Standards Framework (GSF) programme (Thomas 2003a) was notable not only because it offered this approach to cancer patients but that it had the capacity to be extended to all dying patients including people with heart failure.

Central to the delivery of services to the terminally ill in the community is the extension of the best of hospice care out into the community. This means the delivery of care which is the equivalent of the best specialist practitioners but delivered by professionals whose speciality, if you will, is general practice. This 'speciality of the generalist' approach emphasised the importance of improving communication, enabling patients to die where they chose (where possible), 'joined up' assessment of patients' needs, and crucially, the maintenance of the morale of teams doing difficult and demanding work with clients whose needs were ever changing and often unpredictable.

If this success has been visible in the care of cancer patients, can district nurses demonstrate the same success in the care of heart failure patients?

The NICE heart failure guidelines

NICE guidelines

If cancer care has been the subject of numerous public policy initiatives then cardiac care has also benefited from intense scrutiny. Heart failure has, to a greater or a lesser extent, featured as part of this scrutiny. *The National Service Framework for Coronary Heart Disease* (DoH 2000) included a short chapter on heart failure which was welcome as the start of the policy initiatives, but which has also been described by many as being light on detail. Subsequent to this, the National Institute for Clinical Excellence (2003a) fleshed out an approach to patients in heart failure by issuing guidelines which outlined the care a patient might expect as a minimum.

In all, the guidelines amount to ninety-four recommendations. Eight of these are said to be 'key' and are held to be pivotal to the adequate care of patients. District nurses have a responsibility to ensure that as many as possible of these key recommendations are delivered. But some weigh on them more than others. For instance the recommended six-monthly review of stable patients has become a prime district nurses' responsibility. This requires an assessment of a patient's general functioning, fluid management, cognitive status, diet, renal function and medication review. This comprehensive assessment provision is burdensome enough for district nurses with patients already in the community, but the NICE guidelines also recommend that patients previously stabilised in hospital ought to emerge into the community to a primary care team who are fully aware of the management plan for patients. But perhaps the most significant recommendation of the guidelines was that care and management of the patient was for the first time officially declared to be a team effort encompassing the patient as much as the professional staff.

The delivery of these guideline-driven goals is bound to involve difficulties and pitfalls. But many writers including Pateman (2000) have argued that district nurses are in possibly the best place to observe their implementation and to be able to identify shortcomings and areas for improvement early. That said we can say at the outset that considerable work still needs to be done in the fields of education, the preparation of patients for hospital discharge, multi-professional working and supporting patients and carers.

District nurses' role in long-term conditions

Long-term conditions

After all, heart failure is just one of the many chronic diseases that district nurses are already managing in the community. Patients are already and have been since the inception of the NHS kept out of hospital because of the ministrations of district nursing services. Billingham (2003) makes this very point in reviewing the role of district nurses in caring for people with chronic diseases which include diabetes, arthritis, heart failure, chronic obstructive pulmonary disease, dementia and a range of disabling neurological conditions. People with these conditions need professionals with skills in assessment, care management, inter-agency and multi-disciplinary working, and who can orchestrate home care and rehabilitation services. Many have argued that good district nursing is in an ideal position to do this (Goodman *et al.* 2003).

Indeed this argument is further advanced in other major policy statements. In *Supporting People with Long-term Conditions - an NHS and Social Care Model* (DoH 2005b) a vision of an NHS which met patient need at the point of that need was underlined and an appeal was made to break the grip of a service more designed to meet acute crises in large secondary hospitals. In part as the result of importing models of care from US health maintenance organisations, the *NHS Improvement Plan* (DoH 2004b) envisaged moderately complex patients (level II) being managed by district nurses while the more complex (level III) patients would be under the direct supervision of community matrons, chosen for their experience in community management or clinical savoir faire. The express aim here would be the prompt management of the patient's care in the community and the prevention of the patient's condition degrading to the point where acute admission to already overstretched hospitals would be mandated. Already local PCTs have begun to adopt this approach (*Long-term Conditions Strategy*, Southport and Formby PCT 2005).

The most common reasons for referrals for district nursing input are chronic illness, terminal illness, incontinence, wound management and diabetes (Audit Commission 1999). District nurses form the largest single group of employees belonging to the NHS in the community. Already these nurses are the primary point of contact for millions of people with the NHS. However many observers have seen in the district nursing service an underused resource which could be mobilised to take on a much broader and deeper role in the care of patients with these chronic conditions (Arnold *et al.* 2004).

In *Choosing Health* (DoH 2004a) it is argued that nurses have the potential to make a distinct contribution to improve health given their accessibility and local knowledge. District nurses' extensive contacts, particularly with older people, provide a vital source of information. Documenting patients' needs, identifying patients with particular needs, maintaining regimes of investigations, and delivering prophylactic care such as vaccinations could make a real difference in the care of patients with chronic conditions such as diabetes and heart failure.

District nurses' knowledge of heart failure

Knowledge of heart failure

With all of the above accepted, it could still be argued that district nurses have, in common with the rest of the NHS, failed to face up to the enormity of the challenge which has been set by the phenomenon of heart failure. It could be said that this is the result partially of a failure of knowledge: poor understanding of the condition, and a failure of culture: the result of a training which focused on short-term acute recovery rather than long-term chronic management (Gibbon 1994).

Lack of knowledge about the incidence and prevalence of heart failure, of its investigation and likely treatment might incline district nurses to miss the tell tale signs of incipient heart failure among their often elderly and poly-morbid clients. Although it is widely accepted that district nurses deliver to the elderly, with 66 per cent of their nursing delivered to the over-65s (DoH 2002), and although it is accepted that the incidence of heart failure is set to increase by huge numbers, the educational opportunities for nurses in the care of patients with this condition are poorly developed. Less even than such opportunities being offered, there is little knowledge of the training needs of nurses in this field. One American literature study found no research pertaining to this area (Albert *et al.* 2002) and there is little reason to believe that the situation is different in the UK. In fact one is inclined to suspect that more work has been done investigating the learning needs of the patient than the learning needs of the nurse!

In terms of work culture the picture is just as opaque, with both patients and nurses committed to an old fashioned view of district nurses and their roles and responsibilities. With honourable exceptions (Stewart & Blue 2004) little work has yet been done relating to the specific roles of heart failure nurses caring for patients at home, but conclusions drawn from cancer services are hardly encouraging. Luker (2003) for instance found that cancer patients and carers were unsure as to the role of the district nurse. The nurse was ascribed a purely practical role and was only thought likely to visit when physical care such as injections, wound care and infusions were required. This represents an older stereotype which needs to decline if a new model district nursing service is to break through, and patients and carers need to be convinced that a new approach exists based on long-term commitment for patients whose needs will not be immediately resolved (Goodman 2000).

Many of the areas for concern can be illustrated by offering clinical vignettes. Of course the 'patients' so described are fictitious in that they do not exist as individuals. It is the contention of the author however that such patients actually do exist en masse. They are presented as 'before and after' examples of changes made in the region of the author.

Vignette number one

Vignette No. 1

Mary was referred from hospital discharge to the district nursing service for the management of a leg ulcer. The reason for her admission was given as exacerbation of congestive heart failure. No information was given with regard to her prognosis and neither the patient nor her family had any appreciation of the seriousness of her condition. There was confusion around her medication on discharge, which the family were unable to resolve. The hospital pharmacist was contacted and the district nurse was given up-to-date information with regard to the patient's medication and condition. The patient was readmitted to hospital three days later and died.

Commentary

Vignette number one demonstrates an unco-ordinated approach to caring for patients with heart failure and is in striking contrast to a patient dying with cancer who would have been fully informed as to diagnosis and prognosis. Several initiatives have been made in the area where the author works which aim to render the care offered to patients more systematic.

District nurses meet the challenge of heart failure

Organisations responsible for delivering care to patients across the region aim to provide education and training for heart failure and palliative care nurses that will be disseminated among primary care staff. A Gold Standard Framework (GSF) register has been established in each GP practice to include all patients with advanced terminal illnesses. Regular multidisciplinary meetings are planned to update, organise and improve care.

Specialist nurses in non-malignant diseases such as heart failure have been employed to co-ordinate services for patients. Specialist, accredited, heart failure courses at diploma and degree level have been established at local university colleges aimed at health care professionals working in primary care, including district nurses. Primary Care Trusts and District General Hospitals such as Southport and Formby PCT, West Lancashire PCT and Southport and Ormskirk NHS Trust are now working together to develop care pathways and formal discharge referral into primary care services.

The British Heart Foundation (BHF 2003) is using the New Opportunities Fund award of £9 million to fund a network of 76 new heart failure nurse positions across England. The network will help patients retain their independence, provide information and link in with primary and palliative care services.

The following vignette demonstrates the success of initiatives to improve the care of patients with heart failure. Again, this is not meant to be an individual patient, but rather an illustration of what the ordinary patient can expect as 'industry standard' following these reforms.

Vignette number two

Vignette No. 2

Bill was diagnosed with end stage heart failure. Bill and his family were aware of his poor prognosis. His preferred place of care was to remain at home to die. As a patient on the GP practice's GSF register Bill's care management was discussed regularly at the multi-disciplinary team meetings. Supported by the district nursing team, Bill died at home surrounded by his family.

Pippa Witter

The district nurse's role in heart failure management

Nurse's role in heart failure management

It is now accepted as a given that the best management of heart failure patients involves an approach which is multi-disciplinary and draws together the strengths and contribution of differing specialities. The work of Linda Blue *et al.* (2001) has put beyond doubt the positive contribution of nurses in managing heart failure services. This contribution is perhaps most evident in the community. Patient education about the condition and its treatment, home visiting and the early detection of impending problems are all within the purview of the district nursing service. This is arguably mostly the case in residential care homes. Here nurses can supervise the day to day care of patients and ensure that the often complex regimes of medication are maintained. But as well as looking after patients with heart failure, district nurses are in a position to observe the early stages of hitherto undiagnosed heart failure in old people.

Of the other professionals who can make a key contribution to the care of patients is the community pharmacist. They too are an often underused source of advice and expertise and their contribution to medical management of patients is often of the highest importance (Masoudi & Krumholz 2003). The work of Lock (2003) suggests that pharmacists' involvement in management teams can dramatically improve the patients' measured quality of life. The advice of the local pharmacist in the management of patient's questions and problems can make all the difference between a concordant and a non-concordant patient. Lock (2003) describes an initiative in North Hampshire where a unified policy on the care of patients with heart failure developed between the primary and secondary sectors has taken many of these issues to heart.

However it is not only in the area of drug management where district nurses can make a contribution. The nature of heart failure as a 'whole person' condition means that it frequently requires that intervention is called for in the areas of lifestyle. Nutrition, and the avoidance of frank malnutrition, is a key area of advice which the patient can have delivered by the district nurse (Nicol *et al.* 2002 and Pasini *et al.* 2004). The reduction of salt intake, the management of careful fluid balance, the importance of exercise can all be emphasised to patients in the environment in which they are likeliest to remember such advice – in their own homes.

There is a screening tool now available, the Malnutrition Universal Screening Tool (MUST 2004) that is a five-step flowchart for nurses in hospitals, the community and care homes to identify those at risk of malnutrition and to plan an appropriate nutritional support programme. Colonna *et al.* (2003) argue that a complete and continuing education programme for treating heart failure includes an understanding of the causes of the condition, symptoms, diet, salt and fluid restriction, drug regimen, concordance, physical and work activities, lifestyle changes, and measures of self control. These non-pharmacologic treatments can be included in the patient's programme of care and monitored by the district nurse who can then liaise with other health-care professionals in primary care.

Where it has been accepted that the patient is dying of heart failure, it may be considered that the district nurse will have a central role, in exactly the same way as with other fatal conditions such as cancer. Indeed such roles have been put forward as desirable innovations (O'Brien *et al.* 1998). However some caution is called for here. The way in which a death from heart failure unfolds is frequently quite different from that of the cancer patient. In heart failure there can be dramatic remissions of condition, there can be sudden cardiac death and these can compromise any over literal translation of palliative care principles designed for cancer care over to this population. There may be further training requirements to educate and support the nurses involved in this work and the development of deeper collaboration between cardiology and palliative care services to fine tune the care offered to the dying cardiac patient (Hanratty *et al.* 2002).

Cowie (2003) notes that the NICE heart failure guidelines indicate when specialist referral is likely to be necessary, particularly when the diagnosis is in doubt, or when the patient is unwell or failing to respond to standard therapy. However a 'specialist' does not necessarily refer to a consultant cardiologist, but to any healthcare professional with special knowledge and experience in the diagnosis and management of patients with heart failure. This could be a general practitioner with a special interest, a heart failure specialist nurse or a district nurse with the relevant experience and education. The district nursing service could be a vehicle for such interventions.

Collaboration in the management of heart failure

Collaboration

The idea that the dying patient should benefit from the heavy involvement of the district nursing service has met with widespread approval. Hanratty *et al.* (2002) uncovered a most flattering estimation of nurses' abilities in this area given by doctors, particularly in the area of patient communication. Creating a balance between the general practitioners' medical role and the district nurses' caring role is bound to be a source of interesting choices and dilemmas.

In particular it will be interesting to see if the communication between professionals is improved as services for heart failure patients improve. Although there have been several interesting developments in this area it remains a source of patient and carer dissatisfaction and was the subject of adverse comment by the patient representatives on the NICE heart failure guidelines group. (Thomas 2003c) reported that this dissatisfaction with communication was expressed to NICE through their Patient Involvement Unit. 'Communication' in this instance can mean the correct communication between professionals co-ordinating care. However it can have a more sinister meaning. Cowie (2003) suggests that patients with heart failure are offered the sort of euphemistic language which cancer victims were offered thirty years ago. Given the importance of this information, this might at first appear indefensible, but it has an all too human cause. The stop start nature of patients' decline in this condition might not incline a professional to be too graphic in describing the likely fate of the patient as it is, to a degree, unpredictable.

An increased openness about prognosis brings with it growing demands on health professionals and patients who may need psychological support. Doctors often portray themselves as bad prognosticators, admitting that they may accept a poor outlook late in the illness. Nurses, patients and carers, it is suggested, are more realistic predictors (Hanratty *et al.* 2002). The public version of the NICE guideline (*Management of Heart Failure* 2003a) and the subsequent document *Palliative and Supportive Care in Heart Failure* (NHS Modernisation Agency – Coronary Heart Disease Collaborative 2004) should encourage better understanding of the treatment, management and standards that can be expected with regard to heart failure. However, much work needs to be done so that patients and carers feel supported. From the patient's viewpoint a high quality service that is easily accessible is vital with a clear management plan being communicated to patients and their carers.

The way forward

The way forward

Partnership and leadership will be integral to the success of the NICE (2003a) guidelines on heart failure. Health Secretary John Reid speaking to nurse leaders at the chief nursing officers conference stated how he wanted to place caring firmly at the centre of NHS values and encouraged a new generation of entrepreneurial nurses who are willing to take risks, take the initiative and create and implement new ideas (CNO Bulletin 2004). His vision for the future includes nurses winning contracts to provide services under the new General Medical Services contract for general practitioners. Frontline nurses will have opportunities to work in new ways and may wish to extend their current role and range of responsibilities to include chronic disease management (NHS Confederation 2003). In debating the gate-keeping role within primary care services Bigger (2004) believes that primary care nurses are best placed to shape the future of health services provision. Nurses follow protocols, consider practical as well as medical solutions to problems and are fundamentally patient- rather than problem-centred. Potentially, through adoption of the gate-keeping role, district nurses could become the main agent of care for a chronic disease like heart failure. The rational use of nursing skills would enable general practitioners to focus on primary prevention and diagnosis and management of acute illness.

Conclusion

The increased incidence of long-term conditions such as heart failure presents a huge challenge to health professionals. Already highly prevalent in the ageing population, heart failure is likely to increase over the coming years. Much of the onus of caring for the increased patient numbers will fall to health professionals in primary care, especially district nurses.

NICE is not charged with implementing the heart failure guidelines but states that it is up to local health communities to review their existing service provision for the management of heart failure against its recommendations as Local Delivery Plans are developed. There is a genuine willingness to improve the standards of care for heart failure amongst health professionals. With the support of a specialist nurse working across primary and secondary care, the district nurse could be pivotal in reducing hospital admissions by ensuring regular and effective patient contact as recommended by the guidelines.

An educational programme developed especially for nurses in primary care, to provide training on the care of the patient living at home with heart failure could reasonably expect to be as successful as the one in response to the NHS Cancer Plan (DoH 2000b) and the NICE guidance *Supportive and palliative care for adults with cancer* (2004). District nurses have an ability to liaise with other specialities, and communicate with the patients. If the educational initiatives organised by local cardiac networks, university colleges and Primary Care Trusts put support and education in place they will have the confidence to lobby for better discharges from hospital and continued support for patients and carers. The challenge that Thomas (2003b) raised with regard to improving cancer care and to bring the best of the advances made in hospice care out into the community, whilst still affirming the 'speciality of the generalist' in the community, is just as relevant following the *National Service Framework for Coronary Heart Disease* (DoH 2000b) and the NICE guidelines on heart failure (NICE 2003a) and one that district nurses are more than able to deliver.

Note
1. An earlier treatment of this subject was published in February 2005 in the *Nursing Standard,* 19 (24), 38–42, and permission to adapt this chapter has been granted by that publisher..

References

Albert, N.M., Collier, S., Sumodi, V., Wilkinson, S., Hammel, J.P., Vopat, L., Willis, C. & Bittel B. (2002). Nurses' knowledge of heart failure education principles. *Heart and Lung,* 31, 102–11.

Arnold, P., Topping, A. & Honey, S. (2004). Exploring the contribution of district nurses to public health. *British Journal of Community Nursing,* 9 (5), 215–24.

Bigger, M.T. (2004). Debating the gate-keeping role within primary care services. *Journal of Community Nursing,* 18(1), 8–11.

Billingham, K. (2003). Chronic illness challenge. Opinion. *Primary Care NHS Magazine.* April 2003. www.nhs.uk/nhsmagazine/primarycare/archives/apr2003/opinion_Billingham.asp (last accessed: February 7 2005.)

Blue, L., Lang, E., McMurray, J.J.V., Davie, A.P., McDonagh, A., Murdoch, D.R., Petrie, M.C., Connolly, E., Norrie, J., Round, C.E., Ford, F. & Morrison, C.E. (2001). Randomised controlled trial of specialist nurse intervention in heart failure. *British Medical Journal,* 323, 715–18.

British Heart Foundation (2003) *New Opportunities for Health: Heart Failure Networks.* London: BHF.

Bullen, M. (2002). Nursing and cancer care. In *Modernising Cancer Services,* ed. Mark R. Baker. Oxford: Radcliffe Medical Press.

The CNO Bulletin (January 2004) – www.doh.gov.uk/cno/bulletins.htm

Colonna, P., Sorino, M., D'Agostino, C., Bovenzi, F., De Luca, L. & Arrigo de Luca, I. (2003). Nonpharmacologic care of heart failure: counselling, dietary restriction, rehabilitation, treatment of sleep apnea, and ultra filtration. *American Journal of Cardiology,* 91(Issue 9 Suppl.1), 41–50.

Cowie, M.R. (2003). NICE guidelines on heart failure. *Clinical Medicine* 3, 399–401.

Department of Health (1999). *Making a Difference: strengthening the nursing, midwifery and health visiting contribution to healthcare.* London: The Stationery Office.

Department of Health (2000a). *Meeting the Challenge: a strategy for the Allied Health Professionals.* London: The Stationery Office.

Department of Health (2000b). *National Service Framework for Coronary Heart Disease – Modern Standards & Service Models.* London: The Stationery Office.

Department of Health (2000c). *The Nursing Contribution to Cancer Care: A Strategic Programme of Action in Support of the National Cancer Programme.* London: The Stationery Office.

Department of Health (2002). *Statistics and Surveys: District Nursing 2001–2.* London: The Stationery Office.

Department of Health (2003). *The NHS Cancer Plan: Three-year Progress-report – Maintaining the Momentum.* London: The Stationery Office.

Department of Health (2004a). *Choosing Health? A consultation on action to improve people's health.* London: The Stationery Office.

Gibbon, B. (1994). Stroke nursing care and management in the community: a survey of district nurses' perceived contributions in one health authority. *Journal of Advanced Nursing,* 20 (3), 469–76.

Goodman, C. (2000). Exploring the role of the district nurse in rehabilitation. *British Journal of Community Nursing,* 5 (6), 300–4.

Hanratty, B., Hibbert, D., Mair, F., May, C., Ward, C., Capewell, S., Litva, A. & Corcoran, G. (2002). Doctors' perception of palliative care for heart failure: focus study group. *British Medical Journal,* 325 (7364), 581–5.

Lock, J. (2003). The benefits of adding a pharmacist to the heart failure team. *Hospital Pharmacist,* 10 (2), 81–3.

Luker, K.A., Wilson, K., Pateman, B. & Beaver, K. (2003). The role of district nursing: perspectives of cancer patients and their carers before and after hospital discharge. *European Journal of Cancer Care,* 12 (4), 308–16.

The Malnutrition Universal Screening Tool (2004). Available at www.bapen.org.uk

Masoudi, F.I. & Krumholz, H.M. (2003). Polypharmacy and comorbidity in heart failure. *British Medical Journal,* 327 513–14.

NHS Confederation and the National Primary and Care Trust (Nat PaCT) (2003). *The role of nurses under the new GMS contract.* Available at www.nhsconfed.org/publications/gmsbriefing7.asp (last accessed: 7 February 2005).

NHS Modernisation Agency – Coronary Heart Disease Collaborative (2004) *Palliative and Supportive Care in Heart Failure,* NHS Modernisation Agency. Available at www.modern.nhs.uk/chd/documents

Nicol, S.M., Carroll, D.L., Homeyer, C.M. & Zamagni, C.M. (2002). The identification of malnutrition in heart failure patients. *The European Journal of Cardiovascular Nursing,* 139–47.

O'Brien, T., Welsh, J. & Dunn, F.G. (1998). Non-malignant conditions. In Fallon, M. & O'Neill, B. (eds) ABC of Palliative Care. Non-malignant conditions. *British Medical Journal*, **316** (7127), 286–9.

Pasini, E., Opasich, C., Pastoris, O. & Aquilani, R. (2004). Inadequate nutritional intake for daily life activity of clinically stable patients with chronic heart failure. *The American Journal of Cardiology*, **93** (81), 41–3.

Pateman, B. (2000). The changing perspective of caring. *British Journal of Community Nursing*, **5** (6), 264.

Stewart, S. & Blue, L. (2004). *Improving Outcomes in Chronic Heart Failure*. London: BMJ Books.

Southport and Formby Primary Care Trust (2005). *Long-term Conditions Strategy*, 2005/08.

Thomas, V. (2003). Listening to patients helps improve heart failure care. *Guidelines in Practice*, **6** (9), 18.

Bibliography

National Institute for Clinical Excellence (2003a). *Chronic Heart Failure. Management of Chronic Heart Failure in Adults in Primary and Secondary Care*. London: NICE.

National Institute for Clinical Excellence (2004). *Supportive and Palliative Care for Adults with Cancer*. London: NICE.

Cowie, M.R., Wood, D.A., Coats, A.J., Thompson, S.G. *et al.* (2000) Survival of patients with a new diagnosis of heart failure: a population study. *Heart*, **83** 505–10.

Davies, R.C., Bhatia, G., Sosin, M. & Stubley, J., (2003). Barriers to managing heart failure in primary care: heart failure clinics.
Available at BMJ.com/cgi/eletters/326/7382/196

Department of Health (2004b). *The NHS Improvement Plan – Putting People at the Heart of Public Services*. London: The Stationery Office.

Department of Health (2005a). *Improving Chronic Disease Management*. www.dh.gov.uk/PolicyAndGuidance/OrganisationPolicy/PrimaryCare/ (Last accessed: 27 January 2005).

Department of Health (2005b). *Supporting People with Long-term Conditions – An NHS and Social Care Model*. London: The Stationery Office.

Goodman, C., Ross, F., Mackenzie, A. & Vernon, S. (2003). A portrait of district nursing: its contribution to primary health care. *Journal of Interprofessional Care*, **17** (1), 97–108.

Lane, G. (2002). Managing heart failure in nursing and residential care. *Nursing & Residential Care*, **4** (4) 156–60.

National Collaborating Centre for Chronic Conditions (2003). *Chronic Heart Failure: National Clinical Guideline for Diagnosis and Management in Primary and Secondary Care*. London: Royal College of Physicians of London. Available at www.rcplondon.ac.uk

Peterson, S., Rayner, M. & Wolstenholme, J. (2002). *Coronary Heart Disease Statistics: Heart Failure Supplement*. London: British Heart Foundation.

Thomas, K. (2003a). *Caring for the Dying at Home: Companions on the journey*. Oxford: Abingdon, Radcliffe Medical Press.

Thomas, K. (2003b). In search of a good death. Primary healthcare teams in new framework for better care of the dying at home. (Letter to the editor.) *British Medical Journal*, **327** (7408), 223.
Available at http://bmj.bmjjournals.com/cgi/content/full/327/7408/223-a

Chapter 3

The care of patients who develop heart failure alongside mental health problems[1]

Christine Gardner

It scarcely needs to be repeated that the numbers of people who will develop heart disease as the population ages are staggering. But within these figures lie people with heart failure who do not fit the profile of the ageing, post-infarcted patient. There are other, often young, patients who are developing heart failure as the unintended result of treating mental illness. Others may have developed heart failure after living with mental illness for some time. It is the problems of both these groups that this chapter intends to address.

This chapter looks at aspects of care for those patients who have a diagnosis of heart failure but who also may have mental health problems. An article by Gardner and Smith (2004) cites Davidson *et al.* (2001) who describe this type of patient as a 'vulnerable group' whose physical health needs may not be entirely addressed by current practice and management plans, especially when there is a co-existing diagnosis of heart failure.

McKelvie *et al.* (1999) stated that identifying people who are at high risk of heart failure allowed the possibility of implementing strategies that could potentially prevent heart failure and improve prognosis. Patients with mental health problems fall into a poorly recognised category for this type of preventive intervention. Many authors have discussed the reasons why people with mental health problems, such as psychoses and depression, often had their physical health needs overlooked. They are many and varied. The least to be said is that these problems can influence and prohibit thorough investigation into the causes of other health problems including heart failure.

Christine Gardner

A diagnosis of a mental illness can influence a patient's treatment and management, and if this diagnosis is poorly made, then it may have implications for the patient. In heart failure, this could prejudice their ability to obtain treatments most likely to both relieve symptoms and reduce their risk of death (DoH 2000).

Among patients with mental health problems, patients with depression will figure largely, whether this is as a primary condition or as a result of their heart failure. Depression is regarded as a risk factor for the development of ischaemic heart disease. Likewise the response of many patients to the development of heart disease is of profound depression requiring medical treatment.

Shabetai (2002) discusses the presentation of patients' symptoms, which can often be misinterpreted. In heart failure symptoms of fatigue, insomnia, anorexia and palpitations can also be located as diseases of the nervous system. In her article, she wonders whether 'depression should be added to the many conditions that predispose to heart failure'.

In schizophrenia, many of the medications offered to patients (particularly, it must be said, the older variety) can produce Parkinson's Disease type abnormalities of movement (Borders-Hemphill 1998, Keks 1996, Royal Pharmaceutical Society of Great Britain 2002). This can have a profound effect on the patient's ability to attend the doctor's surgery or the hospital. The much trumpeted provision of heart failure clinics and nurse-led services might, for this very reason alone cause the patient with mental health problems to fall from view.

Iatrogenic heart failure

Iatrogenic heart failure

However a more menacing aspect to this problem is the association of these drugs with heart failure, that is to say, in causing heart failure. If one uses the search terms 'schizophrenia' and 'heart failure', in a Cochrane Library search, interesting insights emerge relating to a possible relationship of heart failure with the drug group used for treating schizophrenia.

In a study by Lewis *et al.* (2002) it was revealed that the antipsychotic medication Sertindole was linked to a risk of sudden cardiac death due to disturbances in autonomic dysfunction and was subsequently withdrawn from the market. This might be interesting were one to be considering a drug of this type in a patient with established heart disease. But extend the search to include the words 'myocarditis' and 'cardiomyopathy' and further evidence is revealed. There are numerous papers which refer to the potential for one medication in particular, Clozapine, to trigger cardiomyopathy (Kilian *et al*. 1999, Leo *et al*. 1996).

The propensity of this medication to trigger cardiomyopathy in a population who may already have significant risk of developing cardiac disease obliges health-care professionals to take extra care in the assessment and continuing care of these vulnerable groups. It is not clear that this obligation is being met.

The drug company that manufactures Clozapine (Novartis Pharmaceuticals) had to release alerts (Branswell 2002, Merril *et al*. 2005) stating that all patients with a family history of heart failure should have a cardiac evaluation before being prescribed this drug. This arose from the concern about the possibility of the patients developing myocarditis. This can start off with a mild inflammatory reaction to the drug in myocytes which may, in susceptible individuals, go on to result in congestive cardiac failure.

Drug induced effects mimicking heart failure

Drug induced effects

As heart failure is a syndrome characterised by a reduction in the heart's ability to pump blood around the body (DoH 2000, North Cheshire Collaborative Working Party 2002) there may be a manifestation of several symptoms. Health professionals might expect to see peripheral oedema as one of the common presenting features of patients in heart failure. However, Tamam *et al*. (2002) demonstrated that Risperidone, another atypical antipsychotic drug, may have an association with non-heart-failure-related pedal oedema. It was not clear from the study whether this oedema was due to the drug, or to the deteriorating state of the patients' cardiovascular system, but its potential to introduce confusion in the assessment of mentally ill patients cannot be overlooked.

Christine Gardner

Health-care workers need to be aware of the possibility of this reaction when using this type of medication and identify the problems as they arise, which should then lead to appropriate investigation and treatment, preventing 'assumed' diagnoses of heart failure. The NSF (DoH 2000) itself warns against the possibility of assumed diagnosis arguing that there is also evidence that some people who are treated do not have heart failure.

Patients with mental health problems and risk of cardiac events

Mental health and cardiac risk

Health professionals need to be alert to the possibility of increased cardiovascular risk when using psychotropic medications in this client group. They are also vulnerable to other cardiac events such as ischaemic changes, myocardial infarction, arrhythmias and sudden cardiac death. A particular link with the latter phenomenon was made in an article entitled 'Sudden cardiac death and antipsychotic drugs: Do we know enough?' by Zarate & Patel (2001).

Detecting heart failure

Detecting heart failure

In a paper published in 2000 Khunti *et al.* argued that the use of effective treatment for heart failure relies on the correct diagnosis, and is a key step in the appropriate management of heart failure.

If reporting of symptoms is paramount, then the likelihood of the patient to report symptoms becomes a clinical issue. Rogers *et al.* (2000) indicated that disease specific barriers to communication need to be addressed, and that good communication requires the ability both to listen and to impart relevant information. His study suggests that many heart failure patients make sense of their illness in terms of increasing age and decreasing physical and mental capacities. In the case of mental illness it is possible that patients might not recognise changes in their physical health due to the nature of their psychiatric disorder.

Davidson *et al.* (2001) argued that the mentally ill have unhealthy lifestyles which receive inadequate medical or public health attention. Mental illness is rarely given as a significant risk factor for heart disease. But certain behaviours are so prevalent among this client group that its influence is hard to ignore.

Gardner & Smith (2004) cite the results from the study of Davidson *et al.* (2001), showing that patients with mental health problems could also be identified as having a higher prevalence of smoking including smoking cannabis, obesity, lack of activity and elevated levels of alcohol consumption and salt intake. The latter two are particularly implicated in the development of hypertensive heart failure and cardiomyopathy. They concluded that patients with mental health problems had higher than average risk factors which could expose them to more cardiac disease. This is also supported by studies by Mortensen & Juel (1993), and Herrman *et al.* (1983).

Heart failure and patient co-operation

Patient co-operation

Modern management of heart failure assumes and expects that the patient is compliant with a complex medication regime, changing diets and fluid intake, adapting their activities and monitoring worsening of the condition (Jaarsma *et al.* 1999).

However research studies which examine patient co-operation with treatment frequently exclude people with a co-existing psychiatric condition. Why this is done is not always made clear, though one is entitled to theorise that research teams hypothesise that these patients may not be able to comply with complex treatment regimes and may skew the figures.

In their book, Stewart and Blue (2001) discuss the needs of the elderly who often forget treatment regimes and advice, and also acknowledge 'high risk' patients as *those with the presence of co-morbidity likely to complicate treatment*. As health professionals concerned with cardiovascular care, the treatment and management demands are intense. Nurse-led clinics have developed to help monitor this compliance and adherence (Stewart and Blue 2001).

In heart failure management it is not unreasonable that patients will be taking upward of four drug groups, possibly including ACE inhibitors, beta-blockers, diuretics, digoxin and any other medication they might have had previously prescribed for other conditions. This requires faith in, and understanding of the regime and it has been claimed that polypharmacy in itself could be a reason why compliance breaks down (Corlett 1996).

Seth *et al.* (1990) reported that poor medication compliance poses a significant impediment to effective treatment of a wide variety of illnesses. If medications are to be taken correctly to achieve effective outcomes for improved management, professionals' aim should be directed at ensuring that medication regimes as far as possible are concordant with the patient's own wishes and beliefs, as well as being scientifically valid.

Any person with mental illness being treated by psychotropic medications might find that as well as the complications of these medications, other menacing and cardiotoxic complications may be in store (Reilly *et al.* 2000). In a report published in 2000, Reilly *et al.* reviewed cardiovascular mortality in psychiatric patients and found it to be high in general but especially as the result of drug-induced arrhythmias. They found an increased prevalence of cardiac abnormalities in a schizophrenic population compared with controls and also reported an association with antipsychotic therapy.

It is clear from this that health staff have a fine line to walk. If heart failure symptoms can potentially develop as a direct consequence of psychotropic medication, the obvious first step might be to withdraw the medication, in order to ameliorate the cardiac effects. However, other serious problems might flow from this such as a possible escalation in the patient's psychiatric symptoms.

Leo *et al.* (1996) describe this situation in a case study. In this instance, when the Clozapine was withdrawn due to the development of heart failure, the patient was required to start on diuretics, an ACE inhibitor and anticoagulation therapy, all of which required careful monitoring and biochemical supporting investigations. Unfortunately, her psychiatric symptoms became much worse on withdrawal of the antipsychotic medication. This in turn caused her to be non-compliant with the cardiac medicines.

Feinstein (2002) echoes this evidence and discusses the inability of some psychiatric patients to be able to adhere to cardiovascular recommendations if the underlying psychotic illness is not adequately addressed and managed. This poses a dilemma for both psychiatric staff and heart failure nurses, and underlines the need in these patients for genuinely 'shared care'.

Smith and Henderson (2000) conducted research into information given to patients about the side effects of antipsychotic drugs and found that some side effects were discussed far more frequently than others. Tuunainen *et al.* (2002) reported a review of antipsychòtic medications cited in a Cochrane search. Typical side effects seen with these types of medicines include extra-pyramidal side effects, weight gain, blood disorders, and sexual dysfunction. Warner *et al.* (1996) go so far as to argue that there is a causal relationship between neuroleptic medications and cardiac toxicity but that doctors were relatively unlikely to inform patients of these potentially fatal adverse effects. Awareness of these side effects is essential if health professionals expect compliance with treatment regimes, but there appears to be a lack of awareness even among the professionals coordinating care.

The propensity of psychiatric conditions both to cause and to complicate cardiac conditions raises a batch of training and education questions for doctors and nurses which, at the start of the public health crisis represented by burgeoning numbers of heart failure patients, has barely been discussed let alone met.

Conclusion

The NSF (DoH 2000) demands that we should identify people at high risk of heart failure. There is potentially a huge gap in the service provision for a large group of patients already at high risk in terms of co-morbidity, lifestyle factors and associated drug therapies. Shabetai (2002) puts this succinctly in stating that this is a poorly researched area requiring closer liaison between psychiatrists and cardiologists.

The proper care of these patients requires a genuinely multidisciplinary approach including a mental health contribution to appropriately instigate investigation and treatment, and be able to monitor the condition of these patients in a true 'shared care' approach.

Note
An earlier treatment of this subject was published in November 2004 in *Mental Health Practice*, 8:3 28–30, and permission to adapt this chapter has been granted by that publisher..

Christine Gardner

References

Borders-Hemphill, B.V. (1998). Extrapyramidal symptoms and the elderly. *Journal of American Society of Consultant Pharmacists* (supp.l 4A), **13**, 1–11.

Branswell, H. (2002). Health problems linked by key schizophrenia drug. Canadian press release available at
http://www.canoe.ca/Health0201/21_schizophrenia-cp.htm

Corlett, A.J. (1996). Aids to compliance with medication. *British Medical Journal*, 313, 926-9.

Davidson, S., Judd, F., Jolley, D., Hocking, B., Thompson, S. & Hyland, B. (2001). Cardiovascular risk factors for people with mental health illness. *Australian and New Zealand Journal of Psychiatry.* **35** (2), 196–202.

Department of Health (2000). *The National Service Framework for Coronary Heart Disease* (Chapter Six – Heart Failure). London: The Stationery Office.

Feinstein, R (2002). Cardiovascular effects of novel antipsychotic medications. *Heart Disease,* **4** (3), 184–90.

Gardner, C.M. & Smith, M. (2004). Have a heart: awareness of cardiac problems in mental health patients. *Mental Health Practice,* **8** (3), 28–30.

Herrman, H.E., Baldwin, J.A. & Christie, D. (1983). A record linkage study of mortality and general hospital discharge in patients diagnosed as schizophrenic. *Psychological Medicine*, **13**, 581–93.

Jaarsma, T., Halfens, R., Huijer Abu-Saad, H., Dracup, K., Gorgels, T., van Ree, J. & Stappers J. (1999). Effects of education and support on self-care and resource utilization in patients with heart failure. *European Heart Journal,* **20**, 673–82.

Keks, N.A. (1996). Minimising the non-extra pyramidal side effects of antipsychotics (abstract). *Acta Psychiatrica Scandinavica,* **389** (suppl.), 18–24.

Kilian, J.G., Kerr, K., Lawrence, C. & Celermajer, D.S. (1999).Myocarditis and cardiomyopathy associated with Clozapine. *The Lancet*, **354**, 1841–4.

Khunti, K., Baker, R. & Grimshaw, G. (2000). Diagnosis of patients with chronic heart failure in primary care: usefulness of history, examination and investigations. *British Journal of General Practice*, **50**, 50–4.

Leo, R., Kreeger, J.I. & Kim, K.Y. (1996). Cardiomyopathies associated with Clozapine. *Annals of Pharmacotherapy*, **30** 603–6.

Lewis, R., Bagnall, A.M. & Leitner, M. (2002). Sertindole for schizophrenia (Cochrane review). *The Cochrane Library*, Issue 2, Oxford: update software.
McKee, P.A., Castelli, W.P., McNamara, P.M. & Kannel, W.B. (1971).

Heart failure alongside mental health problems

The natural history of heart failure: the Framingham Study. *New England Journal of Medicine,* 285, 1441–6.

McKelvie, R.S., Benedict, C. R. & Yusuf, S. (1999). Prevention of congestive heart failure and management of asymptomatic left ventricular dysfunction. *British Medical Journal,* 318, 1400–2.

Merrill, D.B., Dec, G.W. & Goff, D.C. (2005). Adverse cardiac effects associated with Clozapine: Review articles. *Journal of Clinical Psychopharma-cology,* 25 (1), 32–41.

Mortensen, P.B. & Juel, K., (1993). Mortality and causes of death in first admitted schizophrenic patients. *British Journal of Psychiatry,* 163, 183–9.

North Cheshire Collaborative Working Party (2002). Heart failure. Cited from unpublished guidelines (2002).

Reilly, J.G., Ayis, S.A., Ferrier, I.N., Jones, S.J. & Thomas, S.H.L. (2000). QT-c Interval abnormalities and psychotropic drug therapy in psychiatric patients. *The Lancet.* 355, 1048–52.

Rogers, A.E., Addington-Hall, J.M., Abery, A.J., McCoy, A.S.M., Bulpitt, C., Coats, A.J.S. & Gibbs, J.S.R. (2000). Knowledge and communication difficulties for patients with chronic heart failure: qualitative study. *British Medical Journal,* 321, 605–7.

Royal Pharmaceutical Society of Great Britain (2002). British National Formulary – Drugs used in psychoses and related disorders. *British National Formularly,* 43 (Anti psychotic drugs 4.2.1), 174–84.

Eisen, S.A., Miller, D.K., Woodward, R.S., Spitznagel, E. & Przybeck, T.R. (1990) The effect of prescribed daily dose frequency on patient medication compliance. *Arch Intern Med.* 150, 1881–4.

Shabetai, R. (2002). Depression and heart failure (Editorial comment). *Psychosomatic Medicine.* 64 (1), 13–14.

Smith, S. & Henderson, M. (2000). What you don't know won't hurt you, (information given to patients about the side effects of antipsychotic drugs). *British Journal of Psychiatry,* 24, 172–4.

Tamam, L., Ozpoyraz, N. & Unal, M. (2002). Oedema associated with Risperidone: A case report and literature review. *Clinical drug investigation,* 22 (6), 411–4.

Tuunainen, A., Wahlbeck, K. & Gilbody, S.M. (2002). Newer atypical antipsy-chotic medication versus clozapine for schizophrenia. *The Cochrane Library* Issue 2. Oxford: Update Software.

Warner, J.P., Barnes, T.R. & Henry, J.A. (1996). Electrocardiographic changes in patients receiving neuroleptic medication. *Acta Psychiatrica Scandinavica,* 93, 311–13.

Zarate, C.A. Jr & Patel, J. (2001). Sudden cardiac death and antipsychotic drugs: Do we know enough? *Archives of General Psychiatry,* **58**, 1168–71.

Bibliography

Bonneux, L., Barendrecht, J.J., Meeter, K., Bonsel, G.J. & van der Maas, P.J. (1994). Estimating clinical morbidity due to ischaemic heart disease and congestive heart failure, the future rise of heart failure. *American Journal of Public Health*, **84**, 20–8.

British Society of Heart Failure (2002). The real-life management of heart failure. *British Journal of Cardiology*, **9**, 8–9.

Carney, R.M., Rich, M.W., Freedland, K.E., Saini J, teVelde,A., Simeone, C. & Clark, K. (1988). Major depression and medication adherence in elderly patients with coronary artery disease. *Psychosomatic Medicine*, **50**, 627–33.

Channer, K.S., McLean, K.A., Lawson-Matthew, P. & Richardson, M. (1994). Combination diuretic therapy in severe heart failure: a randomized control trial. *British Heart Journal,* **71**, 146–50.

Cheshire & Merseyside Cardiac Network (2005). Identification of patients at high risk of cardiovascular disease. Clinical Guidelines 2005.
Accessed at www.cmcn.nhs.uk

CIBIS Investigators and committees (1994). A randomized trial of beta blockade in heart failure. *Circulation,* **90**, 1765–73.

CIBIS-II investigators and committees (1999). The Cardiac Insufficiency Bisoprolol Study (CIBIS II): a randomized trial. *Lancet,* **353**, 9–13.

Coats, A.J.S. (1998). Is preventative medicine responsible for the increasing prevalence of heart failure? *Lancet*, **352** (suppl. 1), 39–41.

Cohn, J.N., Archibald, D.G., Ziesche, S., Franciosa, J.A., Harston, W.E., Tristani, F., *et al.* (1986). Effect of vasodilator therapy on mortality in congestive cardiac failure. *New England Journal of Medicine,* **314**, 1547–52.

Cohn, J.N., Johnson, G., Zieche, S., Cobb, F., Francis, G., Tristani, F. *et al.* (1991). A comparison of enalapril with hydralazine-isosorbide dinitrate in the treatment of chronic congestive heart failure. *New England Medical Journal,* **325**, 303-10.

Corlett, A.J. (1996). Aids to compliance with medication. *British Medical Journal,* **313**, 926–9.

Denollet, J. & Brutsaert, D.L. (1998). Personality, disease severity and the risk of long-term cardiac events in patients with decreased ejection fraction after myocardial infarction. *Circulation*, **97**, 167–73.

Department of Health (2000). National service framework for coronary heart disease. London: Department of Health

Feenstra, J., Grobbee, D.E., Jonkman, F.A.M., Hoes, A.W. & Stricker, B.H. (1998). Prevention of relapse in patients with congestive heart failure: the role of precipitating factors. *Heart,* **80**, 432–4.

Frasure-Smith, N., Lesperance, F. & Talajic, M. (1993). Depression following myocardial infarction. *Journal of the American Medical Association,* 270, 1819–25.

Lief, R.E. & Cline, C.M.J. (1998). Organisation of the care of patients with heart failure. *The Lancet,* **352** (suppl.1), 15–18.

Lief, R.E. & Cline, C.M.J (1998). Heart failure clinics: a possible means of improving care. *Heart,* **80**, 428–9.

McMurray, J.J.V. & Stewart, S. (1998). Nurse led, muti-disciplinary intervention in chronic heart failure. (Editorial). *Heart,* **80**, 430–1.

Packer, M., Bristow, M.R., Cohn, J.N., Colucci, W.S., Fowler, M.B., Gilbert, E.M. *et al.* (1996). The effect of Carvedilol on morbidity and mortality in patients with chronic heart failure US Carvedilol Heart Failure Study Group. *New England Journal of Medicine,* **334**, 1349–55.

Pitt, B., Segal, R., Martinez, F.A., Meurers, G., Cowley, A.J., Thomas, I. *et al.* (1997). Randomized trial of Losartan versus Captopril in patients over 65 with heart failure (Evaluation of Losartan In the Elderly Study, ELITE). *The Lancet,* **349**, 747–52.

Pitt, B., Zannad, F., Remme, W.J., *et al.* for the Randomized Aldactone Evaluation Study Investigators (1999). The effect of spironolactone on morbidity and mortality in patients with severe heart failure. *New England Journal of Medicine,* **341**, 709–17

Rich, M.W., Beckham, V., Wittenburg, C., Leven, C.L., Freedland, K.E. & Carney, R.M. (1995). A multidisciplinary intervention to prevent the readmission of elderly patients with congestive heart failure. *New England Journal of Medicine,* **333**, 1190–5.

Richardson, A., Bayliss, J., Scriven, A.J., Parameshwar, J., Poole-Wilson, P.A. & Sutton, G.C. (1987). Double blind comparison of captopril alone against frusemide plus amiloride in mild heart failure. *The Lancet,* 2, 709–11.

Scottish Intercollegiate Guidelines Network (1999). Diagnosis and treatment of heart failure due to left ventricular systolic dysfunction. Scottish Intercollegiate Guidelines Network.

Stewart, S. & Blue, L. (2004). *Improving outcomes in chronic heart failure.* London: BMJ Books.

Stromberg, A. (1998). Heart failure clinics. (Editorial). *Heart*, 80, 426–27.

The CONSENSUS Trial Study Group (1987). Effects of enalparil on mortality in severe congestive heart failure. Results of the Co-operative North Scandinavian Enalapril Survival Study. *New England Journal of Medicine*, 316, 1429–35.

The Digitalis Investigation Group (1997). The effect of digoxin on mortality and morbidity in patients with heart failure. *New England Journal of Medicine*, 336, 525–33.

The SOLVD Investigators (1991). Effect of enalapril on survival in patients with reduced left ventricular ejection fractions and congestive heart failure. *New England Journal of Medicine*, 325, 293–302.

The Royal Pharmaceutical Society of Great Britain (Working Party) (1997). *From Compliance to Concordance, achieving shared goals in medicine taking*. Publication by the Royal Pharmaceutical Society of Great Britain, with Merck Sharp & Dohme.

Waagstein, F., Bristow, M.R., Swedberg, K., Camarini, F., Fowler, M.B., Silver, M.A., *et al.* (1993). Beneficial effects of metoprolol in idiopathic dilated cardiomyopathy. Metoprolol in Dilated Cardiomyopathy (MDC) Trial Study Group. *The Lancet*, 342, 1441–6.

Weinberger, M., Oddone, E.Z. & Henderson, W.G. (1996). Does increased access to Primary Care reduce hospital readmissions? *New England Journal of Medicine*, 334, 1441-7.

Chapter 4

Adults with congenital heart disease and heart failure

Sarah Ellison

Over recent years there have been many advances in both the surgical and medical management of patients with congenital heart disease. It is largely due to these developments that a relatively new patient group has emerged: adults with congenital heart disease (ACHD). It is estimated that over eighty per cent of children with congenital heart disease are alive at age sixteen (Wren & O'Sullivan 2001). This suggests a growing population and estimates have offered figures of approximately 20,000 adults with complex congenital heart lesions that require specialist care (Somerville 2002). However this specialist care appears to be variable across the UK with only a few nationally recognised centres specialising in the care of this patient group. As these patients get older they can develop further cardiac problems. One of these is heart failure.

When the term heart failure is used images of ischaemic heart disease, hypertension, valve disease and cardiomyopathy come to mind. These are, after all, the major causes of heart failure (McMurray & Stewart 2000) and they can herald a complex collection of problems including cardiac reshaping and rhythm abnormality, exercise limitation and neuro-hormonal activation (Bolger *et al.* 2003). Heart disease of any form can lead to the development of heart failure. Congenital heart disease can be considered one of these diseases. As Ohuchi *et al.* (2003) suggest, ACHD patients often have residual haemodynamic abnormalities and these present problems such as volume and/or pressure overloads which are seen in the more common causes of heart failure. These problems can have significant effects on morbidity and mortality in the later lives of ACHD patients.

The incidence of ACHD patients presenting with heart failure as a late complication of congenital heart disease is increasing (Muhll *et al*. 2004). In considering some of the complex structural abnormalities that can present in congenital heart disease it is hardly surprising that the heart can be placed under huge strain. In many cases of complex congenital heart disease more than one surgical procedure may be required and these may be palliative rather than curative. However it is not just complex abnormalities which may have the hallmarks of heart failure but supposedly simple lesions may also become problematic, an example being that of a repaired atrial septal defect which can still show elevation of natriuretic peptides up to two decades following closure (Bolger *et al*. 2003).

Epidemiology

It is not a straightforward matter to define the numbers of people in the UK who have this problem. What is possible is to calculate the incidence of congenital heart malformations and to multiply this figure by the annual birth rate. Then one can calculate the numbers of people with cardiac lesions who survive to adulthood. This was the approach taken by the Bethesda Conference in the USA (Child *et al*. 2001). One can see easily how the figure generated by this approach has to be regarded as being at best tenuous with a significant potential for error.

But taking these methods as a starting point it has been suggested that as many as 20,000 patients will have had severe congenital cardiac conditions that may now require specialist supervision and care (Somerville 2002).

However the fact that this large group of patients may need specialist care does not mean that they will receive it. Researchers investigating these matters have discovered that many patients with these problems never see specialist care but are rather managed in small general units in district hospitals. That, indeed, is where they are seen if at all (Bowker *et al*. 1998). The depressing suggestion from Bowker's study is that despite the investment in their surgery initially, these are 'lost children'.

Adults with congenital heart disease

Lost, at least, to follow up and specialist after care.

These patients can therefore face a harsh reality. Some of them may go on to develop further cardiac problems, which can in some cases include ventricular dysfunction and symptoms of heart failure. This is likely to be more the case in patients who have the most serious lesions in the first place (Piran *et al.* 2002).

As nurses are increasingly playing a key role in the management of heart failure through nurse-led clinics, we should be prepared for the possible attendance of patients who have ACHD (Adult Congenital Heart Disease). Likewise we should be ready to deal with patients whose demands are often quite distinct from the older aged patient with heart failure and we should be aware of sources of specialist help dedicated to their demands. Finally, we should be aware of the educational and self help infrastructure available to them such as the Grown Up Congenital Heart (GUCH) Patients Association. This intervention alone might help a patient more than any modification of prescription or surgical intervention. The knowledge that one is not alone with these problems can in itself be enormously therapeutic.

Although these patients have special sensibilities and requirements it is still the case that heart failure nurses may have a vital role to play in their care. In common with the older patient the heart failure service provides a bridge between the hospital and community aspects of the NHS. This enables, or can enable, the NHS to deliver 'joined up' care for these patients. It also puts the nurse at the centre of co-ordinating care and mandates the nurse to speak up for the patient when, let us say, communication breaks down. This is not an easy matter for the nurse to deliver well, and it requires skill and sensitivity in the support and counselling offered to the patient.

The patients with the most serious problems may have to seek out the care they need and travel many miles to receive it. Facilities are under resourced and understaffed. For patients with less severe problems they may well be safely managed in District General Hospitals for ongoing care. Although DGHs may not necessarily have ACHD expertise, as long as good communication is maintained with specialist centres and advice and referral can be accessed quickly then they would be able to detect mounting problems and to refer patients appropriately.

The community heart failure nurse could play a key role in bridging the gap between the specialist centres, local District General Hospitals and primary care. This could be in the form of joint working and offering checks between appointments in a community setting. This would ensure that any problems could be identified quickly and appropriate expert advice could be accessed when needed through close communication with specialist centres (Ellison 2006).

The basic principles of caring for patients with heart failure can be applied to both young and older groups. Encouraging health promotion and education, explanation of medication, monitoring for signs of worsening condition, regular blood checks to monitor renal function and counselling regarding any worries or problems that these patients may have. That said there are some problems which apply exclusively to the younger patient. Among these problems the most prominent and the most taxing will be those which relate to job, to mortgage, to travel, to insurance and, possibly the hardest, to relationships and issues such as contraception and pregnancy. Let us tackle this last question first.

Pregnancy

Pregnancy

As the incidence of rheumatic fever has declined, the most common cause of morbidity and mortality from heart disease in pregnancy is due to congenital heart malformations (College of Obstetricians and Gynaecologists 1998). This could be partly due to poor assessment and advice prior to pregnancy and the poor management of these issues during the delivery and post partum period (Somerville 2002). Much of the risks and outcomes of pregnancy within this group are largely dependent on the initial cardiac defect, those most at risk have cyanotic congenital heart disease (Perloff 1991). All congenital heart patients entering into pregnancy are at risk of developing other cardiac complications such as, arrhythmias, heart failure and strokes (Siu, Chitayat & Webb 1999).

From these findings it becomes clear that all (ACHD) patients considering pregnancy should have a full medical and genetic assessment before undertaking it. With careful assessment and planning many patients are able to have a successful pregnancy. Good communication between all professionals is vital, as is seeking expert advice if needed at an early stage.

Contraception

Another important issue for this group of patients is contraception advice. The low oestrogen pill may well be contraindicated in patients at risk of thromboembolism. This would be especially true for those with any degree of heart failure, pulmonary hypertension or cyanosis. Those in heart failure should also be aware of the risks of the morning after pill as this can exacerbate acute fluid retention and/or thromboembolism (Somerville 2002).

Sterilisation, although the most secure method of contraception, is again not without its risks, especially for the group with complex cardiac abnormalities. This method should only be suggested as a last resort. Full discussion with patient, cardiologist, GPs and gynaecologists should be undertaken prior to any decisions being made (Somerville 2002).

Infective endocarditis

Endocarditis is a condition which can affect anybody; however those with congenital heart abnormalities are especially at risk, (Warnes & Deanfield 2001). One of the supporting roles of the heart failure nurse could be to alert the patient to the possibility of this turn of events and to educate them in the signs and symptoms so that prompt treatment can be commenced. There can scarcely be a situation in medicine which rewards early intervention as much as this.

Not only is education required which relates to the signs and symptoms of the disease, but also to activities in life which place the patient at risk of developing it. Dental surgery, body piercing and tattooing are foremost here and may require antibiotic prophylaxis. It goes without saying that any hint of intravenous drug use or any recreational drug use for that matter should be the subject of the most serious warning.

Sarah Ellison

Lifestyle advice

Lifestyle advice

Much of the difficulty that will face this group of patients will not derive from the illness itself but rather from the response of society to their condition. Imagine how frustrating it is, on moving away in young adulthood from the care and protection of parents and family, to find that the route to independence is blocked not by the cardiac lesion but by the building society. A history of congenital heart disease might make life insurance hard to obtain. Loans and mortgages may be no easier to find.

Also, employment difficulties might arise in a patient who needs a lot of time off to travel the length and breadth of the country in search of (rare) specialist services. In fact whole tracts of employment may not be available to a person in this position. It is partly due to these issues that the Grown Up Congenital Heart Patients Association was founded and they offer excellent advice around all these issues and more.

Psychological support

Psychological support

All chronic diseases carry with them a psychological burden. Yet one could argue that as we grow older we, to a greater or lesser extent, come to expect health problems. To be burdened with a chronic illness in youth confounds our idea of fairness and justice and this can easily translate into a 'grief for lost expectations'. This might be a harder problem for those required to care for the patient than the control of physical symptoms.

Of all the chronic illnesses people face it could be argued that heart failure is among the most depressing. There is some evidence that people who have heart failure have a poorer quality of life than those with other medical conditions (Sharpe & Doughty 1998). This view is shared by Adams & Zannad (1998) who found that even those with early stages of heart failure experienced significant impairment with quality of life.

It is hardly surprising that these patients may develop depressive illness when the physical aspects of this syndrome are taken into account. Many patients both young and old with heart failure have what could be described as classic symptoms of the disease, such as fatigue, dyspnoea, swollen ankles and exercise intolerance (Watson *et al.* 2000). This would be difficult for anyone to cope with but it must be especially hard for younger patients who may find it difficult to manage everyday tasks let alone manage to pursue the same levels of activities as their friends. These patients may feel very isolated with their illness and the uncertainty that it may bring to their future; consequently they may need lots of support.

That said, these people have frequently had a lifetime of adjustment to these difficulties and have come to some *modus vivendi* with their condition often mediated by a bleak humour. Nevertheless, the time might come where they need to talk to someone else in their condition. This again is where GUCH Association can be of help through the use of internet message boards and telephone numbers.

For the future, the prospects of this group of patients rest upon the already impressive developments in medical approaches to symptom control. Refined surgical techniques, implantable devices to control arrhythmias, and occasionally heart transplantation or heart lung transplantation (Somerville 2002) are options which may be open to the failing patient. Of course all of these techniques would need to be delivered by a specialist centre experienced in the nature of congenital problems, in the nature of previous surgery and in the inherent risks of reoperation.

Who is responsible for the care of these patients?

Responsibility of care

Young adults with congenital heart disease can develop heart failure and associated cardiac problems. Although efforts to address the growing problem of heart failure have been discussed within the National Service Framework for coronary heart disease (Department of Health 2000) the potential needs of these younger patients fail to be mentioned.

As Hunter (1997) points out there are many difficulties to be addressed for this group. Who, for instance, should take responsibility for their care? They are no longer children so it is not ideal that they remain with paediatricians, however, adult cardiologists have little experience of these patients. The need for specialist centres is ever growing; however only a small percentage may be fortunate enough to access them.

The need for regional guidelines and provision of services for this group has never been greater. Some writers in this field have argued that the fact this class of patients has been cared for by adult cardiologists has led to delivery of sub-standard care. Recommendations for the provision of services have been suggested (Somerville 2002) and these include outreach clinics and a referral system for general practitioners to access specialist centres.

As specialist centres would only need to be few in numbers the role of primary and secondary care heart failure nurses could be a great asset for these patients between appointments. These patients are quite rarely seen but are increasing in numbers. Heart failure nurses need to ensure that when these patients present in clinic they have an understanding of their differing needs in comparison to older cardiac patients.

As this group can be complex it is imperative that those involved in their care are aware of their own professional limitations; however basic monitoring, counselling and education could be given in collaboration with the specialist centres. Registers of heart failure patients in each GP surgery should include details of these patients so they are easily identified and could be given the best care in the most appropriate setting depending on complexity of the initial defect. It is crucial to ensure that rapid access for advice and support from specialist centres is available for both patients and those involved in their care to ensure the best possible treatment can be offered.

Conclusion

As this group grows we need to ensure that our own knowledge and understanding also develops. Perhaps society itself needs to accept that heart disease can affect young people, they warrant equal access to services that are available to other cardiac patients.

It could be suggested that certain types of congenital heart disease are a lifelong condition that deserve the same investment as other diseases, for example diabetes. Many ACHD patients have to pay for their prescriptions, may get abuse for using disabled parking bays and in some cases may have never seen a specialist.

There is a great deal that all health professionals can do for these patients, perhaps simply identifying them in general practice and ensuring that appropriate follow-up care has been received may be a significant starting point.

It goes without saying that further research and education is vital to ensure further understanding of the needs of this group, as is full communication between all members of the multidisciplinary team.

Note
An earlier treatment of this subject was published in January 2006 in *Nursing Times,* 102 (04), 28–31, and permission to adapt this chapter has been granted by that publisher..

Sarah Ellison

References

Adams, K.F. & Zannad, F. (1998). Clinical definitions and aetiology of advanced heart failure. *American Heart Journal*, 135, 5204–15.

Bolger, A., Coates, A. & Gatzoulis, M. (2003). Congenital heart disease: The original heart failure syndrome. *European Heart Journal*, 24, 970–6.

Child, J.S., Collins Nakai, R.L., Alpert, J.S. *et al.* (2001). Bethesda Conference report task force 3 workforce description and education requirements for the care of adults with congenital heart disease. *Journal of American College of Cardiology*, 37, 1183–7.

College of Obstetricians and Gynaecologists (1998). *Why do mothers die? Report on confidential enquiries into maternal deaths in the UK. 1994 1996*. London: The Stationery Office.

Department of Health (2000). *The National Service Framework for Coronary Heart Disease. Heart Failure*. London: The Stationery Office.

Ellison, S. (2006). Challenges in nursing adults with congenital heart disease. *Nursing Times,* 102, 4, 28–30.

McMurray, J. & Stewart, S. (2000). *Epidemiology, aetiology and prognosis of heart failure.* 83, 596–602.

Muhll, I., Liu, P. & Webb, G. (2004). Applying standard therapies to new targets: the use of Ace inhibitors and Beta Blockers for Heart Failure in Adult Congenital Heart Disease. *International Journal of Cardiology*, 97, 25–33.

Ohuchi, H., Takasigi, H., Okada, Y., Yamada, O., Ono, Y., Yagihara, T. & Echigo, S. (2003). Stratification of paediatric heart failure on the basis of neurohormonal and cardiac autonomic nervous activities in patients with congenital heart disease. *Circulation*, 108, (19), 2368–76.

Perloff, J.K. (1991). Pregnancy and congenital heart disease. *Journal of American College of Cardiology*, 18, 340–2.

Piran, S., Veldtman, G., Siu, S, Webb, G.D. & Liu, P.P. (2002) Heart failure and ventricular dysfunction in patients with single or systemic right ventricles. *Circulation*, 105, 1189–94.

Siu, S., Chitayet, D. & Webb, G. (1999). Pregnancy in women with congenital heart defects: what are the risks? *Heart*, 81, 271–5.

Somerville, J. (2002). Grown Up Congenital Heart (GUCH) Disease: current needs and provision of services for adolescents and adults with congenital heart disease in the UK. *Heart*, 88, (suppl. 1), 14.

Sharpe, N. & Doughty, R. (1998). Epidemiology of heart failure and ventricular dysfunction. *The Lancet,* **352**, 13–17.

Watson, R.D., Gibbs, C.R. & Lip, G. (2000). *Clinical features and complications, ABC of heart failure.* BMJ Books, London: Chapter 4, 13–16.

Bibliography

Adams, K.F. & Zannad, F. (1998). Clinical definitions and aetiology of advanced heart failure. *American Heart Journal.* **135**, 5204–15.

Bowker, T.J., Hunter, A.S., Williams, G.J. *et al.* (1998). Does grown up congenital heart disease in district hospitals differ from that in regional cardiac centres? A pilot for a national survey. *Heart.* **79**, (suppl 1), 26.

Cowie, M.R., Mosterd, A., Wood, D. *et al.* (1997). The epidemiology of heart failure. *European Heart Journal*, **18**, 208–25.

Cowie, M.R. (2002). Best practice, evidence from clinical trials. *Heart,* **88**, (suppl. 11), 2–4.

Hunter, S. (1997). Management of adults with congenital heart disease. *Heart*, **78**, 15.

Jolly, L. (2002). The role of the specialist nurse. *Heart*, **88**, (suppl. 2) 33–5.

Jullian, D., Campbell Cowen, J. & McLenachan, J. (1998). Cardiology 7th ed. WB Saunders. 292.

Stewart, S. Mareley, J.E. & Horowitz, J.D. (1999). Effects of a multi disciplinary home based intervention on unplanned readmissions and survival among patients with chronic congestive heart failure a randomized control study. Lancet. 354: 1077 83.

Warnes, C.A. & Deanfield, J.E. (2001). Congenital heart disease in adults. In *Fuster, V., Alexander, R.W., & O'Roarke, R,A, (eds.) Hurst's the Heart,* 10th edn. New York: McGraw Hill, pp. 1907–38.

Wren, C. & O'Sullivan, J.J. (2001), Congenital heart disease. Heart, 85: 438-43.

Zuber, M., Gautschi N, Oechslin, E., Widmer, V., Kiowski, W. & Jenni, R. (1999) Outcome of pregnancy in women with congenital shunt lesions. *Heart*, **81**, 271–5

Chapter 5

Cardiac resynchronisation therapy[1]

Robert Frodsham

There is now almost universal acceptance that heart failure in the western world is the result of damage to cardiac structures which has been wrought by conditions such as ischaemia or hypertension (Cowie *et al*. 2000). The treatment options now open to patients and physicians have expanded beyond all recognition in comparison to even a decade ago.

Yet despite this, and the benefit that millions have derived from such therapies, there are some patients for whom a tightly controlled and regulated regime of ACE inhibition and beta blockade bring little relief. These patients tend to be the more severely ill patients as measured by the New York Heart Association's yardstick of severity – class III or IV. These patients will be subject to the most serious disruption in quality of life (NICE 2003). If that were not enough they will also experience uncomfortable, inconvenient and prolonged admissions to hospital which will cost everybody concerned dearly in terms of money, opportunity costs and human suffering. This is a daunting prospect. The endless cycle of symptoms spinning out of control and ending in ambulance rescue can only count against a patient's psychological adaptation.

Yet, hitherto, the alternatives have been just as stark. Mostly these patients' conditions have slid quickly towards death either from life threatening ventricular arrhythmias or collapse of pump function. The figures for the mortality of these patients are startling even in our day. Studies report a mortality of close to 40 per cent within one year of diagnosis and around 10 per cent each year thereafter (Cowie *et al*. 2000).

However, deeper understanding of the processes which give

rise to these symptoms has led to new approaches to their management. These new therapies rely not on drugs but on electrophysiological manipulation of cardiac activity.

One of the insights into the physiological derangement of heart failure has been the observation of loss of ventricular synchrony. This involves each of the ventricles 'firing' at a slightly different time instead of together. Normally this process is entirely synchronous and results in both ventricles forcing blood against the intraventricular septum and through the pulmonary and aortic valves. Delay in the contraction of either ventricle will manifest itself with an ECG with an extended QRS complex, normally greater than 120 milliseconds. Some studies have suggested that as many as one in three patients with chronic heart failure have evidence of prolonged conduction (Cowie *et al.* 2000). Sometimes this will be in the form of left bundle branch block, often it will not.

The simultaneous contraction of ventricles is lost, usually because the intraventricular septum contracts before either of the ventricles. This dysynchrony compromises the overall efficiency of each contraction.

The net result of this phenomenon is that blood 'swirls' around the ventricle instead of being pushed out. This is particularly so where the ventricles contract while the septum relaxes and vice versa. There is serious compromise of the unified cardiac expulsion of blood which is required for optimum cardiac output. This would be serious enough on its own, but the failure to expel blood results in poor ventricular filling as well as an increased tendency to form blood clots. These will all cause patients' symptoms to deteriorate and could produce other more serious problems such as embolic events.

Cardiac resynchronisation therapy

CRT

As well as loss of synchrony between ventricles, there is in addition the possibility of dysynchrony between the atria and the ventricles. This may affect ventricular filling times and may produce a heartbeat of low efficiency.

Atrio-ventricular dysynchrony was the first clinical situation to be treated by electrophysiological therapies. In the 1980s devices were implanted to reduce the delay between atrial and ventricular contraction. They would stimulate both atrium and ventricle and cause both to contract with an optimum delay between events. It was mainly useful in the treatment of first degree heart block. But for the most seriously ill patients with class III and IV symptoms, there was frequently little or no symptom relief (Gold *et al.* 1995, Linde *et al.* 1995). These patients would have to wait for developments in technology which would permit the pacing of atria and also the pacing of both left and right ventricles. Technically, this was always possible. A transthoracic pacing wire, attached to the left ventricle has always been feasible for patients who have undergone open heart surgery. For the patients who need life long pacing wires, transthoracic approaches are, however, not really a practical solution.

In the 1990s a breakthrough was described which involved pacing the left ventricle using a transvenous approach. Daubert *et al.* (1998) described the placing of a pacing wire over the left ventricle by introducing the pacing wire into the venous system of the heart. This was done by pressing the wire down the coronary sinus and, in a retrograde fashion, along the cardiac veins to overlay the left ventricle. In this way, both the left and right ventricles could be paced and timed with the contraction of the atria. The efficiency of the heart is thus enhanced and heart failure symptoms are reduced. The era of cardiac resynchronisation was born.

Effects of cardiac resynchronisation therapy on cardiac output

Effects of CRT

Resynchronisation therapy works by realigning the contraction of atria and ventricles with each other. But there are other mechanical benefits which accrue to the patient receiving CRT. There is a demonstrable reduction in the degree of mitral valve regurgitation. It has been established that regurgitation of the mitral valve is a common complication of heart failure. It exacerbates symptoms and further reduces cardiac output. This problem is considerably reduced when the ventricles are resynchronised (Etienne *et al.* 2001). Explanations for this phenomenon include alteration in the sequence of ventricular contraction with the timing of the apical and base contraction reversing.

Improving systolic function

Researchers who have investigated the mechanical aspects of cardiac insufficiency have demonstrated by using magnetic resonance angiography that the contraction of the intraventricular septum precedes that of the ventricular wall. This reduces cardiac contractility by producing a 'wobbling' motion in the ventricle, a phenomenon which is clearly visible in severe dilated cardiomyopathy (Curry *et al.* 2000).

The re-establishment of ventricular synchrony attenuates or eliminates this abnormal motion. Cardiac output increases and mean arterial blood pressure increases with it. Not only that, this improvement is accomplished with minimal increase in myocardial oxygen demand. This contrasts sharply with other methods of increasing myocardial efficiency such as inotropic support.

Effects on diastolic ventricular activity

In the normal heart both ventricles fill simultaneously in diastole. Where the left ventricle contracts later than the right ventricle (such as in left bundle branch block), the right ventricle will start to fill before the left. This premature filling might cause the right ventricle to occupy more than its normal share of space in the pericardial sac. If this happens the room for left ventricular expansion may be compromised, and left ventricular output will be reduced. Retiming of the heart by CRT can reverse this process and permit more normal ventricular filling. Optimising ventricular filling in this way will improve myocardial contractility and increase cardiac output.

Clinical trials

All of the above makes sense physiologically. However, the history of medicine is littered with therapies which cannot be translated from the laboratories into practice. Some things may sound as though they will work, but practice can often reveal problems which were unforeseen in the research phase. How, then, has this therapy fared when it has been tried on patients?

Several clinical trials have compared CRT with medical treatment alone, such as diuretic and ACE inhibitor therapy. The Multisite Stimulation in Cardiomyopathies (MUSTIC) study (Cazeau *et al.* 2001) and the Multicenter InSync Randomized Clinical Evaluation (MIRACLE) study (Abraham *et al.* 2002), showed improvements in quality of life, exercise tolerance, NYHA class scores, and left ventricle ejection fraction with CRT.

The MIRACLE study (Abraham *et al.* 2002) also showed a reduction in hospital admissions for worsening heart failure. At six months the risk of admission due to decompensated heart failure reduced by 50 per cent. A 77 per cent reduction in total hospital days saved for treating heart failure was observed in the CRT group compared with the control group.

The COMPANION study (Bristow *et al.* 2000) randomised more than 1,600 patients to medical treatment only, to CRT and to CRT with implantable cardiac defibrillators. The study had to be stopped part-way through because of a 20 per cent reduction in mortality and admission rates in the group with CRT. The group with the most notable benefit, receiving CRT with implantable cardiac defibrillators, showed a 40 per cent reduction in all cause mortality. These preliminary data indicate the benefits CRT may have on mortality.

Possible limitations with this research have to be acknowledged. Many trials have a small sample size, which may undermine the validity of the findings. Trial populations differ from those in clinical practice, for example, older patients and patients with co-morbidities are not well represented, leaving a gap in the evidence. There also appears to be limited follow-up to most trials. However, with the ongoing increase in CRT devices being fitted each year, future studies may be able to provide more answers and guidance for practice.

Psychological considerations

Psychological considerations

The requirement of heart failure patients for high intensity psychological support is well reported. Heart failure may bring in its wake cognitive dysfunction, depression and hypoxia which may all contribute to psychological problems. The insertion of CRT devices complicates this picture further, particularly where they are combination devices which include internal cardioverter defibrillators. This is not uncommon in heart failure where the risk of sudden death by arrhythmia is high. The inclusion of these devices raises still more complex psychological problems (Tagney 2004). In part this question was addressed by NICE in 2000 who acknowledged that implantation and activation of an ICD can cause adverse psychological impact and advocated that people be prepared psychologically for their implantation. While the recognition of this problem was in itself an advance, NICE were less forthcoming about how this might be achieved. Or indeed who was to perform this difficult task. This is one of those fields in which good communication skills will pay immense dividends particularly for nurses in coronary care and cardiology units.

Limitations to the use of CRT devices

Limitations of CRT devices

Given that some studies suggest that up to 20 per cent of patients who receive CRT feel little or no benefit (Reuter *et al.* 2002), one of the limitations of this therapy has to be that selection processes are inexact. Improvements in the selection process will mean less cost and less disappointment for everyone involved. Improvements in particular involving echocardiography may be able to quantify the degree of dysynchrony and offer the possibility of predicting in advance the degree to which a patient will respond to therapy.

That said it is likely that there will always be a degree of failure with this form of therapy. If failure is measured by a reduction in symptoms there may always be people who will not respond. Dyspnoea for instance has many complex causes which may only be marginally improved by CRT. Yet even where the failure to relieve symptoms causes disappointment, there may yet be success in extending life and reducing hospital admissions.

Left ventricular lead placement

Ventricular lead placement

When one considers the occult nature of the coronary venous entrance in the right atrium one ought not to be surprised that there are numerous technical and anatomical problems in lead placement (Daubert *et al.* 1998, Cazeau *et al.* 2001). These difficulties contribute to an estimated 8 per cent fail rate in lead placement. This nearly always affects the left ventricular lead (Abraham *et al.* 2002). Some of the problems relating to lead placement might simply involve difficulty entering the vessel. More serious complications could involve surgical emergencies such as dissection of the cardiac vein. These problems are likely to be reduced as the pool of experienced operators increases.

Conclusion

The interest in CRT has increased over the years and shows little sign of abating. Although the treatment may appear expensive, it would not need many days less hospital admission to justify its cost. Also, the mass production of devices will in time reduce the unit cost of procedures (Bristow *et al.* 2000, Cazeau *et al.* 2001, Abraham *et al.* 2002).

The introduction of new medication regimes and novel management modes such as nurse-led heart failure clinics have all contributed to improved treatment for patients. Further research is required to assess the economic viability of CRT and to determine how it compares to these new regimes and management systems. That said the figures are daunting. If there are 900,000 patients in the UK with heart failure, and up to 30 per cent have wide QRS complexes on ECG, then up to 300,000 patients may need to be considered for CRT. The resources needed to meet those demands are immense and are unlikely to reduce in the foreseeable future.

CRT techniques are becoming more effective with advancements in equipment, facilities and expertise. However, effects on mortality will not be fully determined until further trials are complete. Nurses need to develop their skills and knowledge to provide adequate patient support during informed decision-making regarding CRT and when providing care following resynchronisation.

Note

1. An earlier version of this discussion was published in July 2005 in the *Nursing Standard*, 19, 46–50,and permission to adapt this chapter has been granted by that publisher.

Cardiac resynchronisation therapy

References

Abraham, W.T., Fisher, W.G., Smith, A.L., *et al.* (2002). Cardiac resynchronization in chronic heart failure. *New England Journal of Medicine*, 346, (24), 1845–53.

Bristow, M.R., Feldman, A.M. & Saxon L.A. (2002). Heart failure management using implantable devices for ventricular resynchronisation. Comparison of Medical Therapy, Pacing and Defibrillation in Chronic Heart Failure (COMPANION) trial. COMPANION steering committee and COMPANION Clinical Investigators. *Journal of Cardiac Failure*, 6, (3), 276–85.

Cazeau, S., Leclercq, C., Lavergne, T. *et al.* (2001). Effects of multisite biventricular pacing in patients with heart failure and intraventricular conduction delay. The Multisite stimulation in Cardiomyopathies study. *New England Journal of Medicine*, 344, (12), 873–80.

Cowie, M.R., Wood, D.A., Coats, A.J. *et al.* (2002). Survival of patients with new diagnosis of heart failure: a population-based study. *Heart*, 83, (5), 505–10.

Curry, C.W., Nelson, G.S., Wyman, B.T. *et al.* (2000). Mechanical dyssynchrony in dilated cardiomyopathy with interventricular conduction delay as depicted by 3D tagged magnetic resonance imaging. *Circulation,* 101, (1).

Daubert, J.C., Ritter, P. & Le Breton, H. (1998). Permanent left ventricular pacing with transvenous leads inserted into the coronary veins. *Pacing and Clinical Electrophysiology*, 21, (1 Pt 2), 239–45.

Etienne, Y., Mansourati, J., Touiza, A. *et al.* (2001). Evaluation of left ventricular function and mitral regurgitation during left ventricular-based pacing in patients with heart failure. *European Journal of Heart Failure*, 3, (4), 441–7.

Gold, M.R., Feliciano, Z., Gottlieb, S.S. & Fisher, M.L. (1995). Dual-chamber pacing with a short atrioventricular delay in congestive heart failure: a randomised study. *American Journal of Cardiology*, 26, (4), 967–73.

Linde, C., Gadler, F., Edner, M., Norlander, R., Rosenqvist, M. & Ryden, L. (1995). Results of atrioventricular synchronous pacing with optimised delay in patients with sever congestive heart failure. *American Journal of Cardiology*, 75, (14), 919–23.

National Institute for Health and Clinical Excellence (2000). *Guidance on the Use of Implantable Cardioverter Defibrillators for Arrhythmias*. London: NICE.

National Institute for Health and Clinical Excellence (2003). *Chronic Heart Failure. Management of Chronic Heart Failure in Adults in Primary and Secondary Care. Clinical Guidelines 5*. London: NICE.

Reuter, S., Garrigue, S., Barold S. S. *et al.* (2002). Comparison of characteristics in responders versus nonresponders with biventricular pacing for drug-resistant congestive heart failure. *American Journal of Cardiology*, 89, (3), 346–50.

Robert Frodsham

Bibliography

CONSENSUS Trial Study Group (1987). Effects of enalapril on mortality in severe congestive heart failure: results of Cooperative North Scandinavian Enalapril survival Study (CONSENSUS). *New England Journal of Medicine*, 316, (23), 1429–35.

Cowie, M.R., Wood, D.A., Coats, A.J. *et al.* (1999). Incidence and aetiology of heart failure; a population-based study. *European Heart Journal*, 20 (6), 421–8.

Criteria Committee of the New York Heart Association (1994). *Nomenclature and Criteria for Diagnosis of Diseases of the Heart and Great Vessels*. 9th edn. Boston MA: Little Brown & Co.

Davies, R.C., Hobbs, F.D.R. & Yip, G.Y. (2000). ABC of heart failure: history and epidemiology. *British Medical Journal*, 320, (7226), 39–42.

Dougherty, C.M., Benoliel, J.Q. & Bellin, C. (2000). Domains of nursing intervention after sudden cardiac arrest and automatic internal cardioverter defibrillator implantation. *Heart and Lung*, 29, (2), 79–86.

MERIT-HF Study Group (1999). Effect of metoprolol CR/XL in chronic heart failure: Metroprolol CR/XL Randomised Intervention Trial in Congestive Heart Failure (MERIT-HF). *Lancet*, 353, (9169), 2001–7.

Segev, A. & Mekori, Y. A. (1999). The Cardiac Insufficiency Bisoprolol Study II. *Lancet*, 353, (9161),1361.

Chapter 6

Congestive heart failure and cognitive dysfunction[1]

Joanne Lackey

When a person with heart failure is admitted to hospital in a crisis it is understandable that matters of psychology take a lower priority. After all, staff on cardiology units may not know the person, have little idea of how they were before their heart failure or how their psychological state has been affected by the condition. The priority will inevitably be to save the life of the patient and stabilise their condition.

However the problem with this approach is that the patient's current admission may have been triggered by the very psychological factors which are now falling down the priority list. Poor memory, bad judgement and depression can all contribute to a patient failing to take prescribed medication (Rogers *et al.* 2000). Also failing to remember advice about lifestyle matters such as that about salt and fluid restriction can all result in an emergency admission. In another place I have argued that these factors are often overlooked in the heart failure patient (Lackey 2004). In this chapter I want to argue further that these problems of cardiac dysfunction are first common (Riegel *et al.* 2002) and second currently poorly managed.

Cognition refers to those mental activities associated with thinking, learning and memory (Riegel *et al.* 2002). In all three of these domains people with heart failure can exhibit derangement of function. In one study a team found that problems in all these areas were common in old people with even mild heart failure, defined by a lower than normal ejection fraction (Zuccala *et al.* 1997). This was a finding which was mirrored in younger patients waiting for cardiac transplantation.

They theorised that in the younger group reduced cerebral blood flow was the root of the problem. The problem with the older aged group is that ageing is an independent factor in producing a degree of cognitive dysfunction. People over fifty frequently complain about increasing difficulty with names or numbers. In heart failure these problems are accentuated. One study (Almeida & Flicker 2001) put a figure of 80 per cent on patients with severe heart failure having problems with memory or other mental functions.

This latter study acknowledged the contribution of reduced cardiac output to cognitive dysfunction, but also acknowledged other cardiovascular conditions which could contribute to failing performance. Atrial fibrillation could cause cognitive dysfunction by reducing cardiac output, but it could also do so by the formation and distribution of small clots which cause diffuse brain damage. Valve problems could result in similar effects. Ischaemic heart disease may well be echoed by ischaemic brain disease in an elderly arteriopath and this latter could also cause cognitive dysfunction or even stroke (Almeida & Flicker 2001).

These structural components in the aetiology of cognitive dysfunction are not the only factors which might weigh against the patient's cognitive functions. Other teams have examined broader potential causes of this problem (Riegal *et al.* 2002). The list includes depression, common medical conditions such as chest or urinary tract infections, dehydration and nutritional deficiencies – all common, especially in the elderly. While this list might have a common sense connection with cognitive dysfunction in heart failure it is by no means accepted universally that all of these factors constitute 'smoking guns' for the cause of cognitive problems. Some researchers have argued that the cause of this dysfunction is still obscure. Zuccala (1997) for instance argued that depression was poorly correlated with cognitive dysfunction. Elsewhere Zuccala *et al.* (2005) also argued that the correction of simple metabolic derangement such as blood glucose, electrolytes and haemoglobin paid dividends in the improvement of cognitive function at discharge. The importance of this finding is hard to exaggerate as it suggests that much cognitive difficulty is in fact the result of easily correctable co-morbidities. This in itself is a strong reminder that patients with heart failure require a comprehensive approach to their assessment and treatment (Zuccala *et al.* 2005).

Congestive heart failure and cognitive dysfunction

Other candidates for contributing to cognitive problems include the stasis of blood in the cerebral circulation caused by elevated central venous and right atrial pressures (Riegal *et al.* 2002). Still more include silent cerebral infarcts as well as low intensity cerebral ischaemia. Clotting abnormalities in the elderly may have a role to play here (Taylor & Stott 2002). The importance of describing this 'rogues gallery' of potential causes is to underline that there might be many other causative factors in cognitive dysfunction other than heart failure, even though intuitively it seems obvious that this mechanism will be a leading culprit.

For all its multifactorial aspects the existence of cognitive dysfunction in heart failure patients raises some very demanding questions. Number one, how do these problems impact on patients and carers? In what way do these influences affect mortality and morbidity? How well do the professional services deal with these difficulties? How well are they detected, and where detected, how well are they treated?

The impact on the patient and their carer of cognitive dysfunction

Impact on patient and carer

Moving on from the causes of cognitive impairment, how does this phenomenon reveal itself in patients? Many studies have looked at this question. Some have pointed to complex reasoning skills being compromised (Zuccala *et al.* 1997). Others have highlighted confusion and short-term memory loss (Rogers *et al.* 2000), this being especially relevant in that they affect a patient's ability to communicate and will render a person a 'poor historian'. Antonelli *et al.* (2003) echoed these findings reporting disturbances of verbal functioning which further complicates communication. Other teams have examined how these difficulties affect the ability to maintain complex treatment regimes (Grubb *et al* 2000).

The inability of the person with heart failure to communicate or to engage in complex reasoning, overlying the physical symptoms typical of heart failure can induce the victim to withdraw from physical, social, work and leisure activities. This could itself result in increased depression and anxiety which could reinforce cognitive impairment. It is not hard to see how some writers have suggested that cognitive impairment might lead to increased mortality and morbidity (Almeida & Tamai 2001a). However this view, if correct, carries with it enormous implications. Unassessed and untreated cognitive dysfunction could be costing years of life and increasing the suffering of a vulnerable group. Ethically, this situation is hard to defend.

Screening and treatment – what barriers exist?

Barriers to screening and treatment

New and innovative approaches have been introduced in the management of heart failure patients. It is possible that patients may meet a nurse who will manage their condition. However, this may depend on the patient's address. While the major centres may have such easy-to-access services, other areas may have services which are distant and infrequent and may impose complex travelling arrangements on the patient. Negotiating public transport, walking distances and managing crowded outpatient departments may incline a patient not to bother.

Other problems might be described as more professional in nature. Little agreement exists on how cognitive dysfunction is assessed and managed. The correct beta-blocker might be a matter of professional consensus, but psychological assessment tools? This is especially true of nurses, who are poorly equipped and trained for this type of role.

When differing assessment tools have been examined they have been found to be insensitive to impairment which may be early or fluctuating in severity (Riegal et al. 2002). Yet the fruits of an accurate detection could be enormous. Zuccala (1997) posits that the early detection of cognitive impairment, with prompt intensive treatment of left ventricular systolic dysfunction may prevent or delay a remarkable proportion of dementia in advanced age. Of course it might not. But the whole field raises tantalising questions that only time will give us the answer to. Watson et al. (2000) point out that 'treatment with angiotensin converting enzyme inhibitors prevents or delays the onset of symptomatic heart failure in patients with asympto-matic or minimally symptomatic, left ventricular systolic dysfunction' (p. 329). Would the same be true of heart failure related decline of mental faculties? Or is this too complex a phenomenon to be reduced to a simple problem of failing ventricular performance? Perhaps at the heart of this question are existential matters beyond the scope of chemotherapy. Grubb *et al.* (2000) indicate anxiety, depression and cardiovascular disease as influencing factors. With so many other possible origins of poor cognition it is not entirely clear that maximising heart failure treatment can improve cognition.

If the assessment of cognitive dysfunction is an area fraught with difficulty, then the reversal of such changes is even more difficult. First the studies are few and the numbers studied are low. Almeida and Tamai (2001a) attempted to show that optimising medical treatment over six weeks could improve attention in heart failure patients. In another study in 2001 they suggested that tight management of other illnesses also contributed to improvement in cognition. This makes a sort of common sense (Almeida and Tamai 2001b).

More recently, researchers have attempted to look at new ways of preserving mental faculties and reversing their decline. One group attempted to address the possibility that simple exercise might affect brain function, and initial findings seem to suggest that this might be a possibility along with improving movement speed (Tanne *et al.* 2005).

Assessment and treatment of these problems therefore pose enormous methodological difficulties and, frankly, the data is poor and inconsistent hitherto. How then do patients cope with these difficulties and what support is needed?

Self-management and cognitive dysfunction

Self-management

Where the patient is reeling from the impact of an acute admission, or where the patient is struggling with tissue hypoxia it is difficult enough for the nurse to assess the capacity to consent to treatment let alone understand the complex act of memory required to comply to medical treatment on discharge. Some researchers have advocated the use of patient focus groups to maximise the understanding of the disease and its home management: discussions will improve patients' understanding of the disease and empower them (and their carers) to take a more active role in management (Cowie & Zaphiriou 2002).

Rogers *et al.* (2000) discuss how chronic heart failure patients find it difficult to absorb and retain information and may not appreciate its relevance. They found in their qualitative, interview-based study that patients blamed confusion or short-term memory loss for their inability to ask planned questions of their clinicians. Fatigue also played a major role and many patients were unaware of what heart failure actually was, including their likely prognosis. Lackey (2004) suggests that this inability to remember and assimilate information is contributing to the high readmission rates seen with heart failure. Carlson *et al.* (2001) discuss how self-care is difficult due to the functionally compromised position of the patients. They suggest that patients' knowledge is often poor and misperceptions evident, leading to low confidence and high readmission rates.

With regard to self-management I have highlighted the implications of the above for hospital and community nurses in maintaining stability in these patients (Lackey 2004). A major factor in maintaining stability is medication and lifestyle concordance. Cline *et al.* (1999) assessed compliance to prescribed medication in elderly patients with heart failure. They found that only 55 per cent of patients could correctly name their prescribed medication and 27 per cent were found to be completely non-compliant. It became evident that poor knowledge remains a major issue despite educational initiatives. This underlines the problems facing practitioners in preventing hospital readmissions and managing heart failure in a primary care setting.

The challenge for the NHS is to intervene in the care of heart failure patients and to reverse the cognitive problems caused by falling ventricular performance. This may be an easier problem to describe than to solve. Assessment may be possible but the means of reversing these problems is at an early stage of research.

Implications for the future

Implications

Universally the literature reveals a hard-to-deny link between chronic heart failure and cognitive impairment. However this is an area of heart failure that remains widely unrecognised. 'Often ignored, neurocognitive dysfunction in chronic heart failure represents a daunting morbidity progressing to loss of self-reliance' (Sangha *et al.* 2002). Zuccala *et al.* (2001) highlight the overwhelming challenge it poses to patients, carers and public health services. Although its exact cause remains unclear, the literature advocates early assessment and diagnosis so treatment can be initiated to prevent premature morbidity and mortality. (Almeida & Tamai 2001, Zuccala, *et al.* 2001). It also urges recognition of psychological illness as a common side effect of cardiovascular disease (Grubb *et al.* 2000).

This is an area which is ripe for further research, although the 'pay-back' for research efforts here is frustratingly soft. 'Hard endpoints, such as mortality or days of hospitalisation, are easy to record. Quality of life, disability and cognitive impairment are much more complex and time consuming to measure' (Taylor & Stott 2002). These authors highlight underusage of clinical psychologists in the hospital setting when the causes of heart failure admissions are often psychological in nature. It is not uncommon to see patients known to the service admitted and readmitted because of what is disparagingly referred to as 'acopia', an inability to cope with the demands of daily life. In addition to managing and treating physical and haemodynamic problems, nurses in the acute setting should be assessing mental capability more deeply, initiating prompt referral to specialists when necessary or more realistically, where possible. However time and workload constraints may well make this increasingly difficult. The findings of the studies to date also provide evidence for increased numbers of community heart failure nurses. This will enable screening of patients for impaired cognition and early commencement of appropriate treatment, thus preventing needless hospital admissions. Lackey (2004) highlights that from an ethical perspective, this new aspect of heart failure assessment must be addressed if positive implications for morbidity and mortality can be more definitely confirmed. Riegel *et al.* (2002) agree, 'future research should extend our knowledge about cognitive impairment associated with heart failure by exploring methods of measurement, associated factors and interventions to prevent and manage this problem'.

Note

1. An earlier treatment of this subject was published in July 2004 in the *Nursing Standard,* 8 (44) 33–36 and permission to adapt this chapter has been granted by that publisher.

References

Almeida, O.P. & Flicker, L. (2001). The mind of a failing heart: a systematic review of the association between congestive heart failure and cognitive functioning. *International Medical Journal*, **31**, (5) 290.

Almeida, O.P. & Tamai, S. (2001a). Clinical treatment reverses, attentional deficits in congestive heart failure. *BMC Geriatrics*. **1**, (1), 2.

Almeida, O.P. & Tamai, S. (2001b). Congestive heart failure and cognitive functioning amongst older adults. *Arquivos de Neuro-Psiquiatria*. **59**, (2B), 324–9.

Antonelli, R. *et al.* (2003). Verbal memory impairment in congestive heart failure. *Journal of Clinical Neuropsychology*, **25**, (1), 14–23.

Carlson, B. *et al.* (2001). Self-care abilities of patients with heart failure. *Heart and Lung*, **30**, (5), 1–9.

Cline, C.M., Bjorck-Linne, A.K., Isrealsson, B.Y., Willenheimer, R.B. & Erhardt, L.T. (1999). Non-compliance and knowledge of prescribed medication in elderly patients with heart failure. *European Journal of Heart Failure*, **1**, (2), 145–9.

Cowie, M.R. & Zaphiriou, A. (2002). Management of chronic heart failure. *British Medical Journal*. **325**, 422–5.

Grubb, N. R., Simpson, C. & Fox, K.A. (2000). Memory function in patients with stable, moderate to severe cardiac failure. *American Heart Journal*, **140**, (1), 1–5.

Lackey, J. (2004). Cognitive impairment and congestive heart failure. *Nursing Standard*, **18**, (44), 33–6.

Riegal, B. Bennett, J.A., Carlson, B., Montague, J., Robin, H. & Glaser, D. (2002). Cognitive Impairment in heart failure: Issues of measurement and aetiology. *American Journal of Critical Care*, **11**, 520–8.

Rogers, A.E., Addington-Hall, J.M., Abery, A.J., McCoy, A.S., Bulpitt, C., Coats, A.J. & Gibbs, J.S. (2000). Knowledge and communication difficulties for patients with chronic heart failure: qualitative study. *British Medical Journal*, **321**, (7261), 605–7.

Sangha, S.S., Uber, P.A., Park, M.H., Scott, R.L. & Mehra, M.R. (2002). Difficult cases in heart failure: the challenge of neurocognitive dysfunction in severe heart failure. *Congestive Heart Failure*, **8**, (4) 232–4.

Tanne, D. Freimark, D., Poreh, A., Merzeliak, O. Bruck, B., Schwammenthal, Y., Scwammenthal, E., Motro, M. & Adler, Y. (2005). Cognitive functions in severe congestive heart failure before and after an exercise training program. International. *Journal of Cardiology*, **103**, (2),145–9.

Taylor, J. & Stott, D. (2002). Chronic heart failure and cognitive impairment:

co-existence of conditions or true association? *European Journal of Heart Failure*, **4**, (1), 7–9.

Watson, R.D.S., Gibbs, C.R. & Lips, G.H.Y. (2000). ABC of heart failure: Clinical features and complications. *British Medical Journal*, **320**, 236–9.

Zuccalà, G., Cattel, C., Manes-Gravina, E., Di Niro, M.G., Cocchi, A. & Bernabei, R. (1997). Left ventricular dysfunction: a clue to cognitive impairment in older patients with heart failure. *Journal of Neurology and Neurosurgery and Psychiatry*, **63**, (4), 509–12.

Zuccalà, G., Onder, G., Pedone, C., Cocchi, A., Carosella, L., Cattel, C., Carbonin, P.U. & Bernabei, R. on behalf of the GIFA (SIGG-ONLUS) investigators (2001a). Cognitive dysfunction as a major determinant of disability in patients with heart failure: results from a multicentre survey. *Journal of Neurology, Neurosurgery and Psychiatry*, **70**, (1) 109–12.

Zuccalà, G., Onder, G., Pedone, C., Carosella, L., Pahor, M., Bernabei, R. & Cocchi, A. for GIFA-ONLUS Study Group (2001b). Hypotension and cognitive impairment selective association in patients with heart failure. *Neurology*, **57**, (11), 1986–92.

Zuccalà, G., Marzetti, E., Cesari, M., Lo Monaco, M.R., Antonica, L., Cocchi, A., Carbonin, P. & Bernabei, R. (2005). Correlates of cognitive impairment among patients with heart failure: results of a multicentre survey. *American Journal of Medicine*, **118**, (5), 496–502.

Bibliography

Bennett, S.J. *et al.* (2000). Self-care strategies for symptom management in patients with chronic heart failure. *Nurse Research*, **49**, (3), 139–45.

Department of Health (2000). *National Service Framework for Coronary Heart Disease*, London: The Stationery Office.

Ekman, I., Fragerberg, B. & Lundman, B. (2002). Health-related quality of life and sense of coherence among elderly patients with severe chronic heart failure in comparison with healthy controls. *Heart and Lung*, **31**, (2), 94–101.

Putzke, J.D., Williams, M.A., Rayburn, B.K., Kirklin, J.K. & Boll, T.J. (1998). The relationship between cardiac function and neuropsychological status among heart transplant candidates. *Journal Cardiac Failure*, **4**, 295–303.

Swain, D.G., O'Brien, A.G. & Nightingale, P.G. (1999). Cognitive assessment in elderly patients admitted to hospital: relationship between the Abbreviated Mental Test and the Mini Mental State Examination. *Clinical Rehabilitation*, **13**, (6), 503-8.

Chapter 7

Sexual dysfunction in heart failure

Marj Carey

Introduction

There is now no shortage of evidence available to suggest that quality of life with heart failure is poor and often worse than with other chronic illnesses (Rogers *et al*. 2000). As a result the patient's role within the family, social life and sexual relationships are negatively influenced. This can consequently lead to a further deterioration in quality of life, made worse with the progression of the disease (Cline *et al*. 1999).

The evidence of Westlake *et al*. (1999) suggests that sexuality is an important aspect of quality of life for patients with advanced heart failure and their spouses or partners. Therefore, health care workers involved with patients with this progressive disease should be aware that successful treatment of sexual dysfunction may not only improve sexual relationships but also quality of life.

Working as a cardiac nurse advisor with heart failure patients, I have observed that the subject of sexual activity is rarely broached. Various reasons are given for this. Often there may be embarrassment, lack of awareness and understanding on the subject of sexual dysfunction and of possible treatments that may be available. The author felt that her own lack of knowledge in this area was a barrier to being able to help patients who suffered with this problem. I began to research the subject looking for protocols, guidelines and different approaches to sexual dysfunction in cardiac patients. Drawing from the data available, I concluded that most of the evidence pertained to diabetic and cancer patients and cardiac patients following myocardial infarction (MI) or coronary artery bypass graft surgery. There appeared to be limited information however on sexual dysfunction and the patient with advanced heart failure unless it referred to the pre-transplant period. This suggests that it is not recognised as an issue for the heart failure patient, or given serious consideration as to how this may affect their quality of life or indeed their spouses or partners. Furthermore, whilst searching the data it appears that a diabetic patient can be treated on the National Health Service (NHS) for sexual dysfunction, whereas treatment for the heart failure patient is unobtainable. This is rather surprising, as studies have shown that sexual dysfunction may result from or predict arteriosclerosis (Bernardo 2001).

Therefore, the aim of this chapter is to explore the need for health professionals working with heart failure patients to enquire about their patients' sexual function. It will look at methods of referral, treatment available and it will highlight the barriers that exist for heart failure patients in receiving appropriate treatment. It is hoped that by discussion of such issues health-care workers involved with the heart failure patient will have a greater understanding of the patients' need for information and of the importance of addressing the topic with clients in the future. This will allow them to express any needs or concerns they may have about sexual activity. As a result it is hoped that they may be taken seriously and receive any appropriate treatment that they may require.

Unfortunately, the discussion in this chapter will tend to concentrate on male sexual problems such as erectile dysfunction. The reason for this is that male problems have been the subject of many more studies than female sexual problems. The study of female sexual dysfunction in heart disease is poorly developed. It is not the contention of this chapter that female sexual dysfunction does not exist in heart failure just that the literature is not there for a rounded discussion on the subject. Perhaps this would be a fertile ground for nurse researchers in the future.

Identifying sexual dysfunction

Sexual dysfunction

Arthur (2002) reported that the majority of patients (seventy per cent) suffering with sexual dysfunction are too embarrassed to complain. Furthermore, she states that a further 25 per cent accepted that this was 'a normal part of ageing' and the remainder did not feel that it was 'of particular importance' to them.

Interestingly, fewer than seven per cent of the patients reported that their doctor had actually broached the subject with them. This may seem surprising, given that the availability of oral agents for the treatment of erectile dysfunction has introduced new opportunities for discussion. Yet apparently, this seems to be an area where discussion remains taboo. Westlake *et al.* (1999) found that there was no link between levels of sexual dysfunction and the need for education and counselling. Therefore they advise that health professionals should take the initiative and assume that all patients and their partners require support, counselling and information on this topic.

Sexual problems can be commonplace, affecting a person's mood, close relationships and general health. Erectile dysfunction is the most frequently recognised and readily treated sexual dysfunction (Debusk *et al.* 2000). Erectile dysfunction is reported to affect approximately 30 per cent of men between the ages of forty and seventy years (DeBusk *et al.* 2000). Other less familiar dysfunctions highlighted by Debusk *et al.* 2000) include problems of desire, arousal (both for male and female), orgasm and ejaculation.

Sexual dysfunction in patients with advanced heart failure

Dysfunction in advanced heart failure

The incidence of sexual problems in heart failure is formidably high (Westlake *et al.* 1999). They found that the need for information about sexual problems extended beyond heart failure patients to include their spouses or partners. 75 per cent of the patients reported both a decrease in sexual desire and in the frequency of sexual relations, due mainly, in the patients' view, to their illness. The pathophysiology of heart failure contributes to this sexual dysfunction which deteriorates in line with the deterioration of cardiac function. This will come as no surprise to anyone who cares for a patient in heart failure. Patients who are class III and IV on the New York Heart Association scale will have little inclination for sexual activity.

There is some evidence to suggest that patients following their cardiac transplant have reported that sexual function was amongst ten main areas of their life about which they were least satisfied. They felt that they had been more satisfied prior to the procedure. Of course there could be some severe psychological factors in these problems and some writers have pointed to these factors as a source of sexual difficulties (Bernardo 2001).

Psychological factors may affect sexual dysfunction

Psychological factors

Sexual dysfunction is predominantly treated as a male problem in the literature (Bernardo 2001). However, this is not to suggest that women do not also experience sexual dysfunction. For example if a woman has herself decreased libido it may reduce her motivation in helping her partner regain the capability for satisfying erections. If she has physical barriers to intercourse such as vaginismus which makes intercourse difficult and painful, or vaginal dryness this may increase psychological pressure on her male partner who may already be struggling with impotence as the result of Beta blockade. Penetration failure due to incomplete erection may provoke a high degree of performance anxiety.

Guidelines were produced by four specialists from four different disciplines on the management of erectile dysfunction (Riley *et al.* 2002). According to their guidelines, wherever possible it is advisable to address the sexual disquiet of partners prior to treatment in order to reduce conflict within the relationship. Bernardo (2001) examined the possibility that there may be an intrinsic psychological problem involved in sexual dysfunction. He describes the fear that some patients have about possible failure when sexual activity is resumed such as in patients who have had a myocardial infarction. It is not unusual for patients in this situation to fear that sex may possibly trigger another event. In fact, the risk is very low in patients who have had a myocardial infarction; the possibility of it having been triggered by sexual activity is less than one per cent (Bernardo 2001). Bernardo also states that there are several other factors that influence sexual function such as diabetes, hypertension, obesity and smoking.

Sexual dysfunction in heart failure

Women characteristically complain of loss of libido and genital sensation, vaginal dryness, painful intercourse and difficulty in achieving an orgasm. Other contributing factors for sexual dysfunction in women are previous history of sexual abuse, sexually transmitted diseases or a general feeling of unhappiness and discontentment (Bernardo 2001). A positive influence on sexual activity for the older woman is to have an existing sexually active partner but a negative influence is the presence of concurrent illnesses. Either way, it will do no harm to gently enquire about the possibility of sexual problems among older women. This is not an area without controversy. The author has heard negative comments from both colleagues and patients about older women suggesting that sex is not, and should not be an important issue after a certain age. However, Bernardo (2001) claims that the need for love and sexual activity does not diminish with age or infirmity.

It has now been clearly demonstrated that heart failure patients can experience psychological stress, reduced cognitive function and memory, reduced quality of life and a lack of social awareness (Rogers *et al.* 2000). As a consequence of short-term memory loss, the patient may find it difficult to retain information, and this may prove problematic when giving advice to the patient. As a result of their illness, Rogers *et al.* (2000) reported many patients expressed feelings of anger, depression and anxiety in response to their progressive condition. The higher incidence of depression found among heart failure patients may be in part due to poor communication with members of the multi-disciplinary team (Rogers *et al.* 2000). Furthermore, following their study, Rogers *et al.* (2000) suggested men expressed negativity relating to their condition more than women, and in general older people had reduced expectations regarding their health. Interestingly, heart failure patients have been shown to have the poorest health perceptions compared with those of other patients (Evangelista et al. 2001). Given the significance of this finding, they suggest that routine questioning in general practice could identify erectile dysfunction in diagnosed cardiac patients. Modern therapy can thus be considered in order to restore the sexual relationship in the majority of patients with erectile dysfunction and therefore lead to a substantial improvement in the quality of life. Special care should be given to heart failure patients given their poor health perceptions.

Cardiovascular drugs and sexual dysfunction

Drugs and dysfunction

When talking to patients about their condition it is important to remember that it is not only their condition which will affect sexual functioning. It is also essential to remember the effects of cardiovascular medication on sexual function. 'Antihypertensive drugs, for example, are well known to produce erectile dysfunction, as are some diuretics. Beta-blockers are renowned for causing problems. Cardio-active drugs have the tendency to diminish circulating testosterone' (Jones & Nugent 2001).

The use of beta-blockers has been shown to reduce mortality and morbidity by 35 per cent (Dix 2002). However, a high incidence of sexual dysfunction has been reported with the use of these drugs (Kilgman & Higbee 1989). Across the board iatrogenic, or doctor induced erectile dysfunction is one of the most common presentations of the problem (Kilgman & Higbee 1989).

Angiotensin-converting enzyme (ACE) inhibitors are now universally mandated in heart failure and have been shown to decrease mortality by as much as 25 per cent and also decrease hospitalisation rates (Cowie et al. 2002). In several trials 40 to 80 per cent of patient's experienced an improved functional status when taking ACE inhibitors (DiBianco 1991). However, while many of the drugs taken by heart failure patients improve mortality and morbidity, they can have a detrimental effect on some patients' sex life. Naturally it is more important to ensure that the patient survives before one ensures that their sexual functioning is optimised. Survival, after all, is on the bottom rung of Maslow's hierarchy. The self-actualisation of sexual activity is a desirable feature of this survival but it is not the only one. Additionally, sexual dysfunction can be given additional treatment. Treatment can be tailored to patients' cardiac risk by using (Riley *et al.* 2002) the Guidelines for Management of Erectile Dysfunction of the Princeton Consensus Panel (De Busk *et al.* 2000). This is a simple algorithm to guide physicians in stratifying risk in patients with varying degrees of cardiac disease. Of course it may be that not all erectile dysfunction sufferers may want treatment, and may be just as satisfied with an assessment of their erectile dysfunction or an explanation of the cause.

Risk stratification

When considering referral of heart failure patients for treatment of erectile dysfunction, it is advisable initially to estimate what their usual physical capabilities are (Riley *et al.* 2002). This would therefore determine their capacity for sexual activity without triggering cardiovascular episodes. There are three categories into which all cardiovascular patients fall: low, intermediate or high risk. Ralph and McNicholas (2000) state that the patients with advancing heart failure will fall into the latter grade and therefore will require specialist cardiovascular assessment before treatment for erectile dysfunction can be initiated. They are therefore advised to practice sexual abstinence until their cardiac status has been properly assessed and stabilised, and the cardiologist feels satisfied that there is no risk to the health of the patient in resuming sexual activity. This could provoke negative health perceptions and the health professionals need to deal with this sensitively when aiming to re-establish sexual activity. However, it may be necessary for the cardiologist to refer the patient to a specialised clinic in order to receive appropriate medication and treatment.

The treatment of sexual dysfunction

Impotence has both psychological and physiological aspects, therefore patients will benefit from a more holistic approach to treatment that will take all factors into consideration. Rather than a totally clinical approach it is important to discover the emotional and social needs of the patients. Riley *et al.* (2002) suggests that in order for treatment to be a success resulting in sexual intercourse, the needs of their partners should also be considered. They highlighted the fact that in a group of men seeking treatment for erectile dysfunction, almost half had not experienced any intimate relations with their partners for approximately two and a half years. Therefore, prior to treatment, they recommend that these couples are offered assistance in rediscovering physical intimacy. This may be in the form of a brief explanation regarding sexual function, advice on stimulating techniques and on the role of positive and negative behaviours within a relationship. However, they suggest that some couples may require more intense support via psychosexual or couples therapy. For those patients requiring treatment it is advisable to discuss all options with both the patient and the partner from the outset in order for them to make an informed decision.

Despite the knowledge that diabetes, hypertension and CHD result in this debilitating condition, insufficient consideration is given to erectile dysfunction. In the modern era it is disappointing to note that there are only a few ill-defined references pertaining to sexual activity. The Men's Health Forum and the Impotence Association (2002) found that nearly 90 per cent of people when questioned stated that it is unfair that diabetic men can receive NHS treatment for their erectile dysfunction, whereas those with heart disease cannot. Rules and regulations governing this area may not be as firm as they at first appear. Riley *et al.* (2002) advise that NHS treatment can be considered if the patient is felt to be severely distressed by his erectile dysfunction. Currently there is no evidence that the licensed treatment available for erectile dysfunction adds to the general cardiovascular risk for patients with or without cardiovascular disease (Jackson *et al.* 1999).

Orally acting drugs are very popular with men and their partners and are often used therefore as first line treatment. Licensed treatment includes oral sildenafil (Viagra) and the availability of this drug in primary care has enabled patients to initiate discussion about their sexual function. Of course sildenafil should be used with caution in those men taking nitrate therapy or who have had recent cardiovascular events. Nitrate's propensity to release nitric oxide makes combination with sildenafil likely to cause a dramatic loss of blood pressure. There are other agents which are available to men who may not tolerate sildenafil. There is a sub lingual preparation of apomorphine which has pro-erection properties (Uprima). It has a different mechanism of action in that it increases the sexual 'signals' coming from the brain to the genitals. It is interesting to note that side effects may be experienced when using apomorphine and nitrates, but these effects are substantially less than that observed with sildenafil (Heaton *et al.* 2002). The clinical trials for these drugs differed in outcome assessments so that comparisons about their efficacy are difficult. Research shows that patients should be encouraged to persevere with treatment when using either drug. It has been shown that a higher success rate is achieved with repeated attempts, even if the first few attempts are unsuccessful (Riley *et al.* 2002). Follow-up is paramount in order to obtain optimum management. It needs to be explained to patients that response to any erectile dysfunction therapy will be initially affected by stress, performance anxiety and other factors previously discussed which may inhibit performance. An individual needs to regain confidence and intimacy in the presence of the new drug.

Conclusion

Some general conclusions can be drawn from this chapter. Heart failure is a condition that has a poor prognosis which, according to its severity, has an important impact on the patient's quality of life. This has been shown to affect not only family and social life but also sexual functioning. Furthermore, spouses or partners of the heart failure patient may be affected. It is therefore important for health care professionals to address these factors when implementing interventions with this group of patients. Promoting a return to sexual function may contribute to improvements in the patient's psychosexual adaptation. The health-care professional may need to gain experience and knowledge themselves in order to feel comfortable to discuss sexual issues with heart failure patients. Perhaps the most friendly arena for these discussions is in nurse-led clinics. It could be part of the agenda just like other lifestyle issues. Health-care professionals may assist by using a tactful and sensitive communication strategy where questions regarding sexual functioning are asked. This might highlight a need for further investigation or treatment. It is advisable for health-care profes-sionals dealing with this group to remember that wherever possible the partner should be involved and be encouraged to take part in discussions regarding choices of treatments available. We should assume that the heart failure patient requires information whether or not it is requested. In general we should try to assess changes in the sexual relationship as part of the heart failure evaluation process, taking special care to consider the needs of women and in particular those of the older generation. Moreover, we may counsel patients and their partners about the changes they may experience and attempt to assist them in focusing on ways to cope with their diminishing physical capacity and therefore reduce negative changes which may occur in sexual functioning.

References

Arthur, W.R. (2002). Cardiovascular disorder and erectile dysfunction. *British Journal of Cardiology*, 9 (3), 144–5.

Bernardo, A. (2001). Sexuality in patients with coronary disease and heart failure. *Herz*, 26 (5), 353–9.

Cline, C.M., Willenheimer, R.B., Erhardt, L.R., Wiklund, I. & Isrealsson, B.Y. (1991). Health related quality of life in elderly patients with heart failure. *Scandanavian Cardiovascular Journal*, 33 (5), 278–85.

Cowie, M.R., McIntyre, H. & Panahloo, Z., on behalf of the OMADA investigators. (2002). Delivering evidence-based care to patients with heart failure: results of a structured programme. *British Journal of Cardiology*, 9, 171–80.

Debusk, R., Drory, Y., Goldstein, I., Jackson, G., Kalul, S., Kimmel, S.E., Kostis, J.B., Kloner, R.A., Lakin, M., Meston, C.M., Mittleman, M., Muller, J.E., Padma-Nathan, H., Rosen, R.C., Stein, R.A. & Zusman, R. (2000). Management of sexual dysfunction in patients with cardiovascular disease: recommendation of The Princeton Consensus Panel. *American Journal of Cardiology*, 86, 175–81.

Dix, A. (2002). Managers and Medicine: At the heart of the matter. *Health Service Journal*, March, 33–8.

Evangelista, L.S., Kagawa-Singer, M. & Dracup, K. (2001). Gender difference in health perceptions and meaning in persons living with heart failure. *Heart and Lung*, 30 (3): 167–75.

Heaton, J., Dean, J. & Sleep, D. (2002). Sequential administration enhances the effect of apomorphine SL in men with erectile dysfunction. International Journal of Impotence Research, 14: 61–4.

Jackson, G., Betteridge, J., Dean, J., Hall, R., Holdright, D., Holmes, S., Kirkby, M., Riley, A. & Sever, P. (1999). A systematic approach to erectile dysfunction in the cardiovascular patient: a consensus statement. *International Journal of Clinical Practice*, 53 (6), 445–51.

Jones, C. & Nugent, P. (2001). The problem of erectile dysfunction following myocardial infarction. *Professional Nurse*, 17 (3), 161–4.

Kilgman, E.W. & Higbee, M.D. (1989). Drug therapy for hypertension in the elderly. *Journal of Family Practice*, 28 (1), 81–7.

Ralph, D. & McNicholas, T. (2002). UK management guidelines for erectile dysfunction. *British Medical Journal*, 321, 499–503.

Riley, A., Wright, P., Ralph, D. & Russell, I. (2002). Guidelines for the management of erectile dysfunction. *Trends in Urology, Gynaecology and Sexual Health*, 7 (2), 1–12.

Marj Carey

Rogers, A.E., Addington-Hall, J.M., Abery, A.J., McCoy, A.S.M., Bulpitt, C., Coats, A.J.S. & Gibbs, J.S.R.. (2000). Knowledge and communication difficulties for patients with chronic heart failure: qualitative study. *British Medical Journal*, 321, 605–7.

Westlake, C., Dracup, K., Walden, J.A. & Fonarow, G. (1999). Sexuality of patients with advanced heart failure and their spouses or partners. *Journal of Heart Lung Transplant*, 18 (11), 1133–8.

Mens Health Forum (2002). News release. 'Let's Talk About Sex....' Says Standing Up for Men Campaign, 18/06/2002.
Accessed at: www.menshealthforum.org.uk

Bibliography

Cowie, M.R., Wood, D.A., Coats, A.J.S., Thompson, S.G., Poole-Wilson, P.A., Suresh, V. & Sutton, G.C. (1999). Incidence and aetiology of heart failure. *European Heart Journal*, 20, 421–8.

Department of Health (2002). *National Service Framework for Coronary Heart Disease*. London: The Stationery Office.

Jaarsma, T., Dracup, K., Walden, J. & Stevenson, L.W. (1996). Sexual function in patients with advanced heart failure. *Heart and Lung*, 25 (4), 262–70.

Scottish Intercollegiate Guidelines Network (SIGN). Diagnosis and treatment of heart failure due to left ventricular systolic dysfunction. (February 1999) No.35.

Chapter 8

Exercise training in the management of patients with heart failure
a review of the evidence[1]

Barbara Stephens

Introduction

There is now a widespread and officially recognised place for regular exercise in the rehabilitation of patients with chronic heart failure (CHF). Exercise, once thought appropriate only for patients following myocardial infarction, has broadened out its scope to take in patients with stable heart failure (NICE 2003). It is regarded as a low risk, effective and life enhancing first line management tool for patients in heart failure.

The fall in cardiac output which characterises CHF brings in its wake a complex combination of central and peripheral vascular changes, which, combined with other respiratory and neurohormonal changes, bring an increasing inability to perform physical tasks, dyspnoea and increasing fatigue (Hanson 1994). These are the symptoms which first cause the patient to present and their severity, in the minds of many, better predicts the course of the disease than many formal investigations (Hanson 1994).

'Traditionally trained' nurses may recall that heart failure patients were advised to avoid all types of exercise which, they were told, would 'strain' the heart. Rest and 'taking it easy' was advocated for this group of patients. If the notion of further weakening the heart was not enough to put the patient off, they were also advised more or less expressly that exercise could lead to death by arrhythmia, or a repeat of the damage which first gave them heart failure such as myocardial infarction (Smith *et al.* 1988).

But in the 1980s new ideas relating to exercise began to gain currency. Lack of exercise in the heart failure patient began to be regarded in a similar way to lack of exercise among the rest of the population: that it led to deconditioning, falling functional capacity leading to falling cardiorespiratory reserve and loss of strength and flexibility. Also in the heart failure population it caused changes in blood volume and red blood cell count (Pollack & Schmidt 1995, Clark & Sherman 1998). Not only that, but the rapidly expanding understanding of the pathophysiological events which underpinned the physical changes in CHF led to new and innovative strategies which aimed to arrest or even reverse the physical decline heralded by CHF.

Over the next decade a quiet revolution took place, with the notion gaining hold that, not only was exercise safe for heart failure patients, but was actually beneficial to them and resulted in measurable improvements in exercise tolerance and performance. The previous advice became harder and harder to maintain in the face of growing evidence and by 2003 NICE had issued guidelines marking the final acceptance of exercise in the armoury of those caring for patients in heart failure. This even though its acceptance in principle was not matched with concrete advice on the details of practical implementation of exercise regimes.

Exercise and heart failure

Exercise and heart failure

Towards the end of the 1980s some investigators were able to demonstrate that patients already diagnosed with CHF could improve blood flow and ventilation after a nine month programme of exercise rehabilitation. Subsequent studies demonstrated that carefully selected patients with left ventricular systolic dysfunction (LVSD) who were enrolled in conventional cardiac rehabilitation programmes alongside patients with normal left ventricular function could benefit as much as their colleagues and improve their functional class (Kellerman *et al.* 1988, Kass & Wenger 1988). These initial findings were confirmed by other researchers who demonstrated benefits not only in symptoms, but also in physiological reserve which expands the capacity for exercise (Coats *et al.* 1992). All that was required was the translation of these principles into practice, and the safe application of best techniques into programmes of clinical relevance to patients.

Exercise training: the evidence

Much was still unknown after all about the relative effectiveness of the type, duration and severity of exercise programmes.

Part of the problem with implementing the findings of researchers in the clinical setting has been the correct interpretation of their data. Although the conclusions of research teams seem to confirm that exercise is safe and beneficial it is not immediately clear what beneficial means. Does it mean easier breathing, or does it mean improved skeletal blood flow? Does it indeed mean the more nebulous 'quality of life'? Studies have examined all of these end points. However taking their 'meta-agreement' into account permits us to tentatively conclude that exercise is a good thing for patients and not the threat to life and limb it was once considered to be.

The effects of exercise training in Chronic Heart Failure

Effects of exercise

Given these beneficial effects it is hard to explain the relative paucity of conclusive evidence among CHF patients relating to improvement in left ventricular performance in particular or to improvement in haemodynamic status in general as the result of exercise training in general (Koch *et al.* 1992, Magnusson *et al.* 1996, Sullivan *et al.* 1989, Coats *et al.* 1992, and Belardinelli *et al.* 1995). There is some evidence that participation in exercise programmes attenuates the influence of vaso vagal reflexes and thereby reduces the likelihood of collapse and arrhythmia (Coats *et al.* 1990, 1992). The importance of this finding is hard to exaggerate as it suggests that fears of damaging the patient and exposing them to sudden death might be exaggerated, indeed that patients' risk of sudden cardiac death could be reduced by exercise. No studies have demonstrated a systematic rise in risk of ventricular arrhythmias during exercise training.

An early and profound sign of Chronic Heart Failure is the development of fatigue and limited exercise endurance. This is thought to be caused by poor tissue perfusion which is the result of increased blood vessel resistance and constriction and poor endothelial response, mediated by activation of the sympathetic nervous system and the salt and water retaining action of the rennin-angiotensin-aldersterone (RAA) system (Kao *et al.* 1998,

Drexler 1992). The work of Hornig *et al.* (1996) suggested that blood flow to skeletal muscle could be improved by strength training, such as in the use of weights, which could control and possibly reverse these changes in the pattern of skeletal blood flow.

Another distressing early symptom of heart failure is the development of breathlessness. This may be induced sometimes by minimal exercise and appears to occur even where alterations in blood gases such as oxygen and carbon dioxide are trivial (Sullivan *et al.* 1989). What causes this dyspnoea therefore is a complex interplay of factors involving muscle perfusion and central respiratory drive. Endurance training in the form of walking, cycling or running has been shown to improve the breathing pattern and comfort of subjects, (Meyer *et al.* 1991, Coats *et al.* 1992). Even where derangement of carbon dioxide levels is found to exist and where serum lactate levels indicate poor perfusion of skeletal muscle Meyer *et al.* (1991) found that regular exercise resulted in measurable improvement which, again, resulted in less fatigue.

In terms of quality of life, several studies have attempted to measure this hard to define concept in relation to exercise and the patient with Chronic Heart Failure. The studies performed so far seem to tell a similar story, whether quality of life has been measured by the researcher or reported by the patient. Coats *et al.* (1992) for instance used patients' own reports relating to dyspnoea and fatigue in the performance of activities of daily living to conclude that improvements could be seen in as little as eight weeks on an exercise programme. Koch *et al.* (1992) found similar results. Sullivan *et al.* (1989) on the other hand observed improvements in function measured by the New York Heart Association functional class after a programme lasting 4–6 months. Improvements in quality of life reports should come as no surprise. Locus of control, improvement in symptoms and a can-do disposition are all likely to be enhanced by improving exercise tolerance and physical performance.

Collating the results of all these studies the ExTraMATCH Collaborative (Peipoli *et al.* 2004) were able to establish that exercise was safe and effective in promoting well-being in patients and extending their exercise capacity. They were less clear however on what to recommend in the way of exercise programme, or even the type or duration of such a programme.

Exercise training: the evidence

The type and duration of exercise training

The problem with reviewing exercise programmes is that various studies have looked at degree and duration of these programmes from different perspectives and mean different things by exercise. Certainly all regimes have as their goal the improvement of patients' objectively and subjectively measured function and quality of life (Oana-Eugenia *et al.* 2002). Some studies have examined short periods of intense exercise. Peipoli *et al.* (1996) suggested three times a week for thirty minutes for six weeks. They used short periods of strength training and showed that endurance and exercise tolerance were improved after the programme. However, they commented that this benefit was not sustained and suggested a longer programme of exercise may prove beneficial. Others have suggested longer programmes such as a four times weekly regime lasting twelve weeks (Demopoulos *et al.* 1997). In this study, patients seemed to maintain their benefit over at least six months.

Outside of the confines of a research laboratory however, it is hard to see the clinical application of such a programme. In a world where space on a rehabilitation programme is at a premium such an intense programme would of necessity have an upper limit on eligible numbers. An alternative approach examined a self-administered programme relying on patients supervising their own exercise patterns at home (Hambrecht *et al.* 1997). This approach also demonstrated that patients could improve their muscle response and oxygen uptake. The difficulties of such a programme are easy to imagine. In the absence of peer pressure, self supervised patients would be inclined, especially on 'bad days' to give themselves time off the programme. In other words, if compliance fell to below 60 per cent the improvements became unmeasurable.

Throughout the literature authors have agreed that patients with Chronic Heart Failure should undertake some form of exercise training more than three times a week, for between 30 and 60 minutes each session (Sullivan *et al.* 1989, Meyer et al. 1991, Koch *et al.* 1992, Belardinelli *et al.* 1995 and Demopoulos *et al.* 1997). The length of the programmes however differed in duration from three weeks (Meyer *et al.* 1991) to thirteen weeks (Koch *et al.* 1992).

The overall opinion is that a longer period of exercise shows better results (European Society of Cardiology Task Force 2001).

The type of exercise to choose is a little complicated. In the majority of studies endurance (constant) cycle training or interval (short periods of exercise between periods of rest) training is employed to improve overall aerobic capacity. Whereas other authors preferred strength training using light weights on either individual or consecutive muscle groups (Monotti *et al.* 1990, Hornig *et al.* 1996, Gordon *et al.* 1996) or in some cases a combination of local strength and endurance was employed (Magnusson *et al.* 1996)

Jones and West (1995) identify that the most common form of exercise used is the treadmill. Not only do cardiology departments have such items in stock, but they involve a familiar type of exercise – walking. Not only that but walking is also an activity of daily living and will be useful to the, predominantly elderly, person in their day-to-day life.

That said the other type of exercise used in experiments, the cycle, can be controlled by the patient who frequently feels safe and secure from falling while on the machine (Williams 1994). The trouble is that cycling may use muscle groups unfamiliar to the patient and these may tire more easily than other muscle groups.

For patients who may become easily exhausted Thompson *et al.* (1997) put forward the advantages of interval training which enables the patients to take extended recovery periods between bursts of activity.

Other studies have eschewed endurance programmes for strength programmes. These are particularly useful among the more seriously ill patients who cannot tolerate endurance exercise for any extended periods. In this group patients exercise individual muscle groups and thereby reverse the effects of deconditioning. It has been suggested that such exercises can increase blood pressure (Magnusson *et al.* 1996) but the extra demands placed on the heart are not thought to be excessive.

Again in reality, the demands of the patient's life are likely to require a degree of endurance (walking to the shops) and strength (carrying shopping). Concentrating on one type of activity to the exclusion of the other, it could be argued, prepares the patient poorly for real life. Meyer *et al.* (1991) argue that patients' exercise programmes should be individually tailored and should combine both elements for three times a week over eight to ten weeks. Other authors have also emphasised the importance of warming up and cooling down exercises.

Of course there will always be some patients for whom no exercise programme will be advised. These will include patients with significant obstructive valvular disease such as aortic stenosis, viral or auto-immune myocarditis and exercise induced arrhythmias. They will be advised not to undertake any form of exercise. In addition, patients with unstable coronary disease or decompensating heart failure should be stabilised prior to exercise training. These patients apart, it is remarkable how few patients exist for whom there are absolute contraindications. Patients with heart failure should be offered exercise in a similar way to any other patient with heart disease. The most important point is to establish the cause of the patient's Chronic Heart Failure and any other limitations before they participate in a programme (Clark & Sherman 1998, Kao & Jessup 1998). Unlike patients who sustain an uncomplicated myocardial infarction and who exercise in a standard class, the patients with Chronic Heart Failure should have their exercise individually prescribed and tailored to their limitations and desired level of activity. This programme should incorporate the type of activity they should undertake at home.

Establishing an exercise training programme

Establishing exercise training

The research therefore all seems to point in the same direction, even if it does so in an inconsistent and heterogeneous fashion. Exercise, however defined, confers on patients psychological and functional benefits, however defined. But before any programme of exercise is implemented there are practical details to be considered.

There are the obvious issues to take account of, the 'where' and the 'whens' and the 'what withs'. An interesting issue arises with the 'who'. For however safe this might be regarded as a form of therapy it is essential that one member of staff is on hand who is skilled in advanced life support just in case the worst should come to pass. Indeed the entire programme should be supervised by a nurse or physiotherapist who has experience and training in dealing with high risk cardiac patients. The prescription of exercise should be regarded as a matter of skill as it requires the tailoring of regimes to the individual's condition. All staff should be skilled in basic life support and how to observe warning signs.

Because these patients are considered 'high risk' (i.e. have an increased chance of cardiac arrhythmias or arrest) the exercise sessions should involve a maximum of eight to ten patients with a ratio of three patients to one member of staff. This is to ensure that patients are closely supervised and are exercising effectively and safely. Most of the patients in the studies had an average age of 60 years, but in 'real life' many patients with Chronic Heart Failure are over 70 years of age (Clark *et al.* 1998). Therefore the results of the studies do not translate directly into clinical practice. Owen and Croucher (2000) have more recently exercised patients over the age of 75 years with no problems. They concluded that elderly patients tolerated appropriate exercise and this resulted in improvements in exercise tolerance.

In addition, most patients with Chronic Heart Failure have developed a degree of sedentary life and they often have co-morbidities, such as chronic respiratory disease, diabetes or renal impairment, that may contribute to their inactivity (Meyer *et al.* 1991). The patients may be fearful of undertaking increased activity, worried about worsening their condition. They may not have exercised for many years and may be apprehensive of coming to a gymnasium and using equipment, wearing casual clothes and not achieving the expected outcome. As part of the educational component of the programme the issues surrounding exercise should be addressed. These are all issues that health professionals need to be aware of in an attempt to overcome both physical and psychological barriers to the change in lifestyle.

To overcome any apprehension the whole professional team needs to support the concept of exercise training. Senior members, including consultants and general practitioners need to be in full agreement concerning its benefits. Should the patients receive any negative comments from a doctor they may well be reluctant to participate.

Before commencing any form of exercise, patients should undergo a physical assessment. This would include a history of their recent health to note any deterioration in their health status, in particular breathing, and peripheral oedema or chest pain. Blood pressure and heart rate should be recorded as a baseline measurement and repeated at each exercise session. One study has recommended using the Minnesota Living with Heart Failure Questionnaire (MLHFQ), a reliable and valid self-assessment quality of life tool, as a predictor of worsening symptoms (Rector *et al.* 1987). This could be employed as a method of assessing patients in addition to other aspects of the assessment.

To assess patients for exercise and exercise prescription there are simple non-invasive, objective methods to determine patients' initial level of fitness. The six-minute walk test is easily accessible, valid and reliable for patients with CHF (Shah *et al.* 1998). This entails patients walking between two fixed spots for six minutes and the distance they cover in those six minutes is then measured as a baseline assessment.

Once an individualised plan has been prescribed the patients can then be taught the series of exercises, how to use any equipment and how to employ a rating of perceived exertion scale (RPE). The RPE is a subjective method the patients use to determine how hard they are working. Using a Likert scale of 6–20 the patient can score his or her level of exercise and is able to assess the effort required during the exercise training. For example if the patient scores 6 they are working very very lightly, if they score 19 they are working very very hard. On average patients should be scoring between 10 and 15. This method of assessment has proved useful in both healthy subjects and those with chronic illness (Thompson *et al.* 1997).

As with all exercise, before the patient begins the exercise training they should undertake a warm-up period. In general, this usually takes 10–15 minutes with healthy subjects; with patients with Chronic Heart Failure this should take at least 20 minutes (Smart *et al.* 2003). During the session patients should be monitored for side effects of exercise including chest discomfort, breathlessness and light-headedness. If this occurs they should be told to inform a member of staff who will assess the situation and treat as necessary. The session should end with a prolonged 'cool down' similar in length to the warm up.

Barbara Stephens

Assessment and evaluation of exercise training

Evaluation of exercise training is a crucial aspect of the programme and can be undertaken in a number of ways. If the MLHFQ was employed this would assess whether patients' quality of life had improved over time. Owen and Crocher (2000) used this method but saw no significant changes in score. Yet Shah *et al.* (1998) use the same scoring and showed significant improvements following exercise training.

The six-minute walk test could be undertaken at the end of the programme and this would also evaluate the effectiveness of the programme. The aim would be to see an improvement in performance with regards to the distance achieved within the time frame. Another aspect of evaluation could be a review at six months to establish if the patients had maintained a more active lifestyle and maintained a degree of improved fitness.

Conclusion

This review of literature regarding exercise training for patients with Chronic Heart Failure concurs with the NICE guidelines and follows the commonly held belief that exercise training improves exercise tolerance and symptoms of Chronic Heart Failure. It supports the view that exercise is both physically and psychologically beneficial to patients with Chronic Heart Failure. In addition, from a practical point, it can be concluded that exercise training is relatively safe and from the research the appropriate methods of exercise together with the frequency and duration can be established.

However, there are much broader issues surrounding the development of this type of exercise programme for patients with Chronic Heart Failure, not least the need to secure funding to develop this new and extensive service. To achieve this within the NHS there needs to be more extensive research that confirms that exercise training is not only beneficial to the individual patients with Chronic Heart Failure, but is foremost a cost effective method of managing this already overwhelming and expensive illness.

Note
1. An earlier treatment of this subject was published in April 2004 in the *British Journal of Nursing*, 13 (8) 452, and permission to adapt this chapter has been granted by that publisher.

References

Clark, J.R. & Sherman, C. (1998). Congestive Heart Failure: training for a better life. *The Physician and Sports Medicine*, 26 (8), 11–17.

Coats, A.J.S., Adamopoulos, S., Meyer, T.E., Conway, J. & Sleight, P. (1990). Effects of physical training in chronic heart failure. *Lancet*, 335, 63–6.

Coats, A.J.S, Adamopoulos, S., Radelli, A., McCance, A., Meyer, T.E. & Berbardi, L., *et al* (1992). Controlled trial of physical training in chronic heart failure. *Circulation*, 85, 2119–31.

Demopoulos, I., Bijou, R., Fergus, I., Jones, M., Strom, J. & LeJemtel, T.H. (1997). Exercise training in patients with severe congestive heart failure: enhancing peak aerobic capacity while minimising the increase in ventricular wall stress. *Journal of American College of Cardiology*, 29 (3), 597–603.

Drexler, H. (1992). Skeletal muscle failure in heart failure. *Circulation*, 85, 1621–3.

European Society of Cardiology Task Force (2001). Guidelines for the diagnosis and treatment of chronic heart failure. *European Heart Journal*, 22, 1527–60.

Hambrecht, R., Fiehn, E., Neibaier, J., Weigl, C., Hilbrich, L., Adams, V., Riede, U. & Schuler, G. (1997). Effects of endurance training on mitochondrial ultra structure and fiber type distribution in skeletal muscle of patients with stable chronic heart failure. *Journal of American College of Cardiology*, 29 (5), 1067–73.

Hanson, P. (1994). Exercise testing and training in patients with chronic heart failure. *Medicine and Science in Sports and Exercise*, 26 (5), 527–37.

Hornig, B., Maier, V. & Drexler, H. (1996). Physical training improves endothelial function in patients with chronic heart failure. *Circulation*, 93, 210–14.

Jones, D. & West, R. (1995). *Cardiac Rehabilitation*. London: British Medical Journal Publishing.

Kao, W. & Jessup, M. (1998). Exercise testing and exercise training in patients with congestive heart failure. *Journal of Heart Lung Transplant*, 13 (4), 117–21.

Kellerman, J.J, Shemesh, J. & Ben-Ari, E. (1988). Contra-indications to physical training in patients with impaired ventricular function. *European Heart Journal*, 9, 71–7.

Koch, M., Douard, H. & Brouster, J.P. (1992). The benefits of graded physical exercise in chronic heart failure. *Chest*, 101 (suppl. 5), 231–5.

Magnusson, G., Gordon, A., Kaijar, J., Syven, C., Isberg, B. & Karpakka, J. (1996). High intensity knee extensor training in patients with chronic heart failure. Major skeletal muscle improvements. *European Heart Journal*, 17, 1048–55.

Barbara Stephens

Meyer, T.E., Casadei, B., Coats, A.J.S., Davey, P.P., Adamopoulos, S. & Radaelli, A. (1991). Angiotensin-converting enzyme inhibitor and physical training in congestive heart failure. *Journal of International Medicine*, 230, 407–13.

Monotti, J.R., Johnson, E.C., Hudson, T.L., Zuroski, G., Murata, G. & Fukushima, E. (1990). Skeletal muscle response to exercise training in congestive heart failure. *Journal of Clinical Investigation*, 86, 752–8.

National Institute for Clinical Excellence (2003). *Chronic Heart Failure: Management of Chronic Heart Failure in Adults in Primary and Secondary Care.* London: NICE.

Oana-Eugenia, S.C., Teodorescu, C.M., Dam, M., Tache, G., Gurun, M. & Dorobantu, M. (2002). Exercise training and left ventricular function in patients with heart failure. *Journal of American College of Cardiology*, 26, (Suppl. May) 235.

Owen, A. & Croucher, L. (2000). Effects of exercise in elderly patients with heart failure. *European Journal of Heart Failure*, 2, 65–70.

Peipoli, M., Clark, A.L., Volterani, M., Adamopoulos, S., Sleight, P. & Coats, A.J.S. (1996). Contribution of muscle afferents to haemodynamic, autonomic and ventilatory responses to exercise in patients with chronic heart failure. *Circulation*, 93, 940–52.

Peipoli, M. *et al.* (2004). Exercise training meta-analysis of trial in patients with chronic heart failure. (ExtraMATCH). *British Medical Journal*, 328, 189.

Pollack, M. & Schmidt, D.H. (1995). *Heart Disease and Rehabilitation* (3rd edn.) New York: Human Kinetics.

Rector, T.S., Kubo, S.H. & Cohn, J.N. (1987). Patients' self-assessment of their congestive heart failure: II. Content, reliability and validity of a new measure – the Minnesota Living with Heart Failure Questionnaire. *Heart Failure*, 3, 198–209.

Smart, N., Fang, Z.U. & Marwick, T.H. (2003). A practical guide to exercise training for heart failure patients. *Journal of Cardiac Failure.* 9 (1), 49–58.

Smith, T.W., Braunwald, E. & Kelly, R.A. (1988). The management of heart failure. In *Heart Disease*, Braunwald, (ed.) Philadelphia: W.B. Saunders.

Sullivan, M.J., Higginbottom, M.B. & Cobb, F.R. (1989). Exercise training in patients with chronic heart failure delays ventricular anaerobic threshold and improves sub maximal exercise performance. *Circulation*, 79, 324–9.

Thompson, D.R., Bowman, G.S., De Bono, D.P. & Hopkins, A. (1997). *Cardiac Rehabilitation.* London: Royal College of Physicians.

Williams, M.A. (1994). *Exercise Testing and Training in the Elderly Cardiac Patient.* Philadelphia: Human Kinetics.

Bibliography

Belardinelli, R., Berman, N. & Purcaro, A. (1995). Exercise training improves left ventricular diastolic filling inpatients with dilated cardiomyopathy. *Circulation*, 91, 2775–84.

Department of Health (2000). *The National Service Framework for Coronary Heart Disease*, London: The Stationery Office.

Gordon, A., Tyni-Lenne, R., Persson, H., Kaijser, L., Hultman, E. & Sylven, C. (1996). Markedly improved skeletal muscle function with local training in patients with chronic heart failure. *Clinical Cardiology*. 19 (7), 568–74.

Kass Wenger, N. (1988). Left ventricular function. Exercise capacity and activity recommendations. *European Heart Journal*, 9, 63–6.

Shah, N.B., Der, E., Ruggerio, C., Heindenreich, P.A. & Massie, B.M. (1998). Prevention of hospitalisation for heart failure with an interactive home monitoring program. *American Heart Journal*, 135, 373–8.

Sullivan, M.J., Higginbottom, M.B. & Cobb, F.R. (1988). Exercise training in patients with severe left ventricular dysfunction. *Circulation*, 78, 506–15.

Chapter 9

Exercise
The things we don't know

Michelle Kerr

There have been countless reviews of the beneficial effects of exercise training in heart failure but very few articles discuss the uncertainties surrounding the subject. In an attempt to redress the balance, the author will highlight these issues.

One of the most notable features of long-term reduction in cardiac output is the emergence of circulatory, peripheral, neurohormonal, respiratory and skeletal changes. These changes may cause symptoms of fatigue and breathlessness, often leading to exercise intolerance (Watson *et al*. 2000). This can be defined as the loss of ability to move large muscle masses due to fatigue or breathlessness (Pina *et al*. 2003) and is largely due to an inadequate blood flow secondary to impaired cardiac output (Sullivan & Cobb 1992).

The management of heart failure has changed dramatically over recent years. Although the introduction of medication such as ACE inhibitors has seen a reduction in symptoms and mortality (The AIRE Study Investigators 1993), there are other treatments which may help to improve the patient's quality of life. In addition to nurse specialist intervention and increased patient involvement, exercise training has been found to improve functional capacity and reduce side effects in selected patients with chronic heart failure (Braith & Thompson 2002). In view of similar research, the SIGN Guidelines (SIGN 2002) recommend a programme of exercise for stable patients. Specific guidelines are not provided as to the details of such exercise programmes, as the direct effects of varying exercise regimes are still uncertain. Also uncertain is the ideal duration, frequency, mode and intensity of training (Meyer *et al.* 1997). The NSF (Department of Health 2001) for coronary heart disease also supports the inclusion of exercise in cardiac rehabilitation.

The concept of exercise training in heart failure has not always been universally accepted. In as late as 1989, Braunwald (1989) argued that 'Reduced physical activity is critical in the care of patients with heart failure throughout their entire course'. However, there is very little scientific evidence to support this statement, with few documented studies on rest therapy. Two trials by Burch *et al.* (1963) suffered a greater than 50 per cent death rate in patients who were kept on long-term bed rest. Surprisingly, earlier research had demonstrated a significant decrease in heart size in 11 out of 36 patients with cardiomegaly with bed rest but it must be recognised that 11 people in these trials went on to die from thromboembolic complications (Burch *et al.* 1963).

In our day, exercise is thought to have a positive effect on chronic heart failure patients. Studies have shown training to improve exercise capacity (Coats *et al.* 1992), subsequently resulting in a comparable improvement in quality of life (Herz *et al.* 2001). In addition, benefits have been reported in muscle structure and in the physiological response to exercise, such as enhanced endothelial function (Hambrecht *et al.* 1998) and improved oxygen extraction at the peripheries of the circulatory system (Pina *et al.* 2003).

Despite the benefits of exercise training in heart failure for most people, it must be recognised that exercise can trigger in a sub-group of patients both sudden cardiac death and more frequently, an acute myocardial infarction (Morantz 2003). 'It is known that approximately 4 to 20 per cent of myocardial infarctions occur during or soon after exertion' (Morantz 2003). Many of the controversial issues surrounding exercise training in chronic heart failure shall now be discussed.

Intensity, mode, frequency and duration

Optimum training mode

The optimum training mode for patients in heart failure has not yet been identified but the majority of studies have included a treadmill or stationary cycle (Pina *et al.* 2003). A select few have undergone interval training, which alternates intensive exercise with easy, slow activity – particularly useful in patients with marked exercise intolerance (Belardinelli *et al.* 1999). Squires (1998) also emphasises the benefits of activities such as walking, as opposed to cycling, to develop the muscles which will be used in daily activities of living. However the overall health improvements associated with any aerobic exercise must not be overlooked (Berg-Emons *et al.* 2003).

Again there has been large variation in the frequency of training programmes. Belardinelli *et al.* (1999) found an improvement in patients' condition following exercise with a frequency of two to three times per week. Hambrecht *et al.* (2000) client group on the other hand underwent twenty minutes of exercise per day. Many other studies however, fail to provide details on the precise duration of exercise undertaken.

The time scale of exercise programmes also varies dramatically. Niebauer *et al.* 2005) found benefits after just eight weeks, whilst Hambrecht *et al.* (1998) and Belardinelli *et al.* (1999) undertook six and twelve month studies respectively. Sustained benefits on discontinuing exercise are also unclear, as functional capacity has not been reassessed at a later date (Pina *et al.* 2003).

As is apparent, the ideal intensity, mode, frequency and duration of exercise training in heart failure remain unclear (Meyer *et al.* 1997). Until there is clarification an individualised approach is essential (Fletcher *et al.* 2001).

Resistance training

Although training programmes have traditionally emphasised aerobic exercise, some researchers have pointed to a beneficial relationship between resistance training and health (Pollock *et al.* 2000). Through the repetitive lifting of light weights, resistance training offers development of endurance and muscular strength – essential in many activities of daily living. Hare *et al.* (1999) found no deterioration in symptoms with resistance training in nine chronic heart failure patients. On the other hand although there was no improvement in the rate of the body's oxygen consumption, there was an increase in strength and endurance. In an attempt to clarify the rationale for resistance training, the AHA Science Advisory published 'Resistance Training in

Individuals With and Without Cardiovascular Disease' (Pollock *et al.* 2000). Even within this document, there is little evidence to support the benefits of resistance training in heart failure. It is highlighted that patients with poor LV function may develop serious ventricular arrhythmias or wall-motion abnormalities and therefore only patients who can achieve more than five or six metabolic equivalents without angina or ST segment changes, should be considered for resistance training. As many heart failure patients are unable to train at such a level, it is unlikely that resistance training will be combined with aerobic activity for the majority of clients.

Ventricular remodelling

Ventricular remodelling

Following a myocardial infarction (MI), the heart muscle undergoes a dynamic process of remodelling, which can affect the size and shape of the left ventricle (LV) (Pina *et al.* 2003). Over the last few years, the influence of exercise training on myocardial wall thinning has generated much debate (Braith & Thompson 2002). Research has provided mixed results on the subject. A non-randomised, controlled study of patients after an anterior myocardial infarction compared the deterioration in ejection fraction between an exercising and a non-exercising group. The patients who had completed twelve weeks of exercise had a significantly greater drop in ejection fraction than the control group (Jugdutt *et al.* 1988). In contrast Cannistra *et al.* (1999) reported variable results in ventricular dilatation in patients following myocardial infarction who were subject to an exercise programme. Some had a reduction in size, others an increase, while some patients remained unchanged. Different conclusions were suggested in a study by Hambrecht *et al.* (2000). This study was restricted to patients with chronic heart failure. His results were more encouraging, demonstrating a small decrease in LV end diastolic diameter and volume. It should be recognised however, that the studies were undertaken prior to the wide use of beta-blockade. They are also relatively small studies and are difficult to compare, due to the variation in client groups: presenting condition, age, sex etc. These factors cast some doubt as to whether the findings may be generalised to other heart failure patients.

Exercise: the things we don't know

Catecholamine release

Catecholemine release

Raised plasma catecholamine levels are thought to be a predictor of poor outcome in chronic heart failure (Watson *et al.* 2000). Following a reduction in cardiac output, neurohormonal systems are activated to preserve circulatory homeostasis (Clark & McMurray 2001). In heart failure long-term sympathetic activity leads to continued catecholamine release, and this brings in its wake a progressive decline in circulatory performance. It was hoped that exercise training would contribute to the reduction in catecholamine release but studies in this area have proved inconclusive. Tyni-Lenne *et al.* (2001) identified that following a three month programme of exercise, patients experienced a reduction in catecholamine levels when compared to a non-exercising group. This was further supported by a similar trial over a six month period by Kjaer *et al.* (2003). However Keteyian *et al.* (1999) did not find any change in catecholamine levels. It must be recognised once again that the above trials were all small in size. There was marked variation in both the sample groups and the exercise programmes undertaken, making it difficult to interpret data with any accuracy.

Mortality

Mortality

Despite an increasing interest in the benefits of exercise training in chronic heart failure, there is still little known as to the effect on mortality. In an attempt to clarify the situation, the ExTraMATCH Collaborative (2004) performed a meta-analysis of nine datasets, totalling 801 patients with left ventricular dysfunction. It was found that although the mechanism was unknown, survival time was significantly increased. The study however does raise some questions. Reported mortality data sometimes differed from that in the initial study. One trial had a considerably larger reduction in mortality than the others but was unidentifiable from the other studies, therefore preventing further scrutiny. Finally one-third of the trials could not provide data regarding medication changes, therefore casting doubt on the influencing factors in survival. In view of these findings, further, more sensitive research would be required to confirm the outcome.

Michelle Kerr

Valvular disease and heart failure

It is known that severe stenotic or regurgitant valve disease is a contraindication to exercise in heart failure patients (SIGN 2001). However this exclusion does not apply to mild to moderate cases, even though there is no supporting data on the efficacy or safety of exercise training among these patients (Pina *et al.* 2003). On the contrary, Rosen *et al.* (1994) found that patients with ventricular dilatation failed to increase left ventricular ejection function during exercise. This may lead to an increase in symptoms and further deterioration of the mitral valve (Pina *et al.* 2003). Of similar concern, is the knowledge that patients with apparently normal valves on echocardiogram, can develop structural changes of the mitral valve to accommodate myocardial remodelling (Grande-Allen *et al.* 2005). This can cause dilatation of the mitral annulus during exercise and therefore induce regurgitation (Pina *et al.* 2003). Consequently stroke volume is reduced, as is cardiac output. Stevenson *et al.* (1990) claim that this can be attenuated by reducing after load through the use of diuretics and vasodilators. Once again it must be noted that many patients are now treated with beta-blockade, an agent not routinely in use when the majority of studies were undertaken. Following a literature search, the impact of exercise-induced mitral regurgitation does not appear to be well documented. It is unlikely to be taken into account therefore, during risk stratification for exercise in heart failure. It may also offer one explanation as to why the functional capacity of some patients is less than might otherwise be expected.

Diastolic dysfunction

Some researchers have argued that up to 40 per cent of heart failure in patients occurs where ventricular systolic function is normal, but where there is a failure of the muscle in diastole to relax properly and that it is abnormal filling of the ventricle that produces symptoms (Davie *et al.* 1997). This condition is known as diastolic dysfunction and is usually the consequence of age, ischaemia or hypertrophy (Davie *et al.* 1997). The management of this phenomenon is based on control of the physiological factors that are known to affect ventricular relaxation – blood pressure, heart rate, blood volume and myocardial ischaemia (Aronow *et al.* 1990). Exercise has been shown to exert a positive outcome on several of these factors and so may be beneficial for such patients (Pina *et al.* 2003). Levy *et al.* (1993) found that LV diastolic dysfunction associated with the ageing process was less pronounced in elderly long distance runners, when compared to age-matched sedentary individuals. However, all of the study participants were in good health and the trial did not address the issue of exercise training as a treatment for diastolic dysfunction. There have also been several studies involving the intense physical training of rats (Bowles & Starnes 1994). Results demonstrated an enhanced cardiac output during hypoxic conditions. These findings however are only found as a result of intense training and as many heart failure patients have at least a degree of exercise intolerance, they may be unable to achieve a level of exercise which may facilitate conditioning. Despite the knowledge that there are no definitive clinical trials in this area, endurance exercise training is still recommended (Morantz 2003).

Tentative conclusions

It is apparent from the issues raised, that there are numerous problems related to the research into exercise training and heart failure. The most obvious is that of sample size. All the trials are small in number and even meta-analysis does not produce credible figures. This makes it difficult to conclude that any improvements in condition are due to the exercise itself and casts doubt on whether findings can be generalised to other patients with chronic heart failure. Of a similar nature is the choice of client group. Many of the studies did not include women or the elderly population and therefore did not test the hypothesis that benefits would also apply to these groups, intensity, mode, frequency and duration of exercise again reducing the value of data collected. It must also be recognised that the trials were undertaken prior to the widespread use of beta-blockade and it is therefore debatable as to whether the benefits of exercise would be in addition to this therapy. Finally, as patients with heart failure will naturally fluctuate between functional classes, it is difficult to determine whether deterioration in condition is due to the variability of symptoms or due to the exercise itself (Hambrecht *et al.* 1998).

While the physical and psychological benefits of exercise are hard to deny, the detail of rehabilitation programmes for patients for heart failure is hard to sketch out. The research evidence for the type, duration and intensity of exercise is still elusive, and only large and well controlled investigations will clarify some of the most tantalising questions.

Exercise: the things we don't know

References

Aronow, W.S., Ahn, C. & Kronzon, I. (1990). Prognosis of congestive heart failure in elderly patients with normal versus systolic function associated with coronary artery disease. *American Journal of Cardiology,* 66,1257–9.

Belardinelli, R., Georgiou, D., Cianci, G. & Purcaro, A. (1999). Randomised, controlled trial of long-term moderate exercise training in chronic heart failure. *Circulation,* 99, 1173–82.

Berg-Emons, R., Balk, A., Bussman, H. & Stam, H. (2003). Does aerobic training lead to a more active lifestyle and improved quality of life in patients with chronic hart failure? *European Journal of Heart Failure,* 6, 95–100.

Bowles, D.K. & Starnes, J.W. (1994). Exercise training improves metabolic response after ischemia in isolated working rat heart. *Journal of Applied Physiology,* 76 (4), 1608–14.

Braith, R.W. & Thompson, P.D. (2002). Exercise for those with chronic heart failure. Matching programs to patients. *The Physician and Sportsmedicine,* 30 (9), 29.

Braunwald, E. (1989). *Heart Disease.* Philadelphia: WB Saunders Co.

Burch, G.E., Walsh, J.J. & Black, W.C. (1963). Value of prolonged bed rest in management of cardiomegaly. *Journal of the American Medical Association,* 183, 81–7.

Cannistra, L.B., Davidoff, R., Picard, M.H. & Balady, G.J. (1999). *Journal of Cardiopulmonary Resuscitation,* 19 (6), 373–80.

Clark, A.L. & McMurray, J.J.V. (2001). *Heart Failure. Diagnosis and Management.* London: Martin Dunitz Ltd.

Cline, C.M., Willenheimer, R.B., Erhardt, L.R., Wiklund, I. & Isrealsson, B.Y. (1999). Health-related quality of life in elderly patients with heart failure. *Scandanavian Cardiovascular Journal,* 33 (5), 278–85.

Coats, A.J., Admpoulos, S. & Radaelli, A. (1992). Controlled trial of physical training in chronic heart failure: exercise performance, haemodynamics, ventilation and autonomic function. *Circulation,* 85, 2119–31.

Davie, A.P., Francis, & C.M. Carvana, L. (1997). The prevalence of left ventricular diastolic filling abnormalities in patients with suspected heart failure. *European Heart Journal,* 18, 981–4.

Department of Health (2001). *National Service Framework for Coronary Heart Disease.* London: The Stationery Office.

ExTraMATCH Collaborative (2004). Exercise raining meta-analysis of trials in patients with chronic heart failure. *British Medical Journal*, **328**, 189.

Fletcher, G.F., Balady, G.J. & Amsterdam, E.A. (2001). Exercise standards for testing and training: a statement for healthcare professionals from the American Heart Association. *Circulation*, **104**, 1694–1740.

Grande-Allen, K.J., Borowski, A.G. & Troughton, R.W. (2005). Apparently normal mitral valves in patients with heart failure demonstrates biochemical and structural derangements. *Journal of the American College of Cardiology*, **45**, 54–61.

Hambrecht, R., Fiehn, E. & Weigl, C. (1998). Regular physical exercise corrects endothelial dysfunction and improves exercise capacity in patients with chronic heart failure. *Circulation*, **98**, 2709–15.

Hambrecht, R., Gielen, S., Linke, A. & Fiehen E. (2000). Effects of exercise training on left ventricular function and peripheral resistance in patients with chronic heart failure: A randomised trail. *Journal of American Medical Association*, **283** (23), 3095.

Hare, D.L., Ryan, T.M. & Selig, S.E. (1999). Resistance exercise training increases muscle strength, endurance and blood flow in patients with chronic heart failure. *American Journal of Cardiology*, **83**, 1674–7.

Haskell, W.L. (1994). Health consequences of physical activity: understanding and challenges regarding dose-response. *Medicine and Science in Sports and Exercise*, **26**, 649–60.

Herz-Kreislauf-Zentrum Gernsbach/Schwarzwald (2001). Exercise and muscle strength training and their effect on quality of life in patients with chronic heart failure. *European Journal of Heart Failure*, **4** (5), 627–34.

Jugdutt, B.I., Michorowski, B.L. & Kappagoda, C.T. (1988). Exercise training after anterior Q wave myocardial infarction: importance of regional left ventricular function and topography. *Journal of American College of Cardiology*, **12**, 362–72.

Keteyian, S.J., Brawner, C.A. & Schairer, J.R. (1999). Effects of exercise training on chronotropic incompetence in patients with heart failure. *American Heart Journal*, **138**, 233–40.

Kjaer, A., Appel, J., Hildebrandt, P. & Petersen, C.L. (2003). Basal and exercise-induced neuroendocrine activation in patients with heart failure and in normal subjects. *European Journal of Heart Failure*, **6** (1), 29–39.

Levy, W.C. Cerqueirs, M.D., Abrass, I.B., Schwartz, R.S. & Stratton, J.R. (1993). *Circulation*. **88** (1), 116–26.

Meyer, K., Gornandt, L., Schwaibold, M., Westbrook, S., Hajric, R. & Peters, K. (1997). Predictors of response to exercise training in severs chronic congestive heart failure. *American Journal of Cardiology*, **80**, 56–60.

Exercise: the things we don't know

Morantz, C.A. (2003). AHA releases statement on exercise and heart failure. *American Family Physician*, **68** (5), 969.

Niebauer, J., Clark, A.L., Webb-Peploe, K.M., Boger, R. & Coats, A.J. (2005). Home-based exercise training modulates pro-oxidant substrates in patients with chronic heart failure. *European Journal of Heart Failure*, **7** (2), 183–8.

Pina, L.I., Apstein, C.S., Balady, G.J., Belardinelli, R., Chaitman, B.R., Duscha, B.D., Fletcher, B.J., Fleg, J.L., Myers, J.N. & Sullivan, M.D. (2003). Exercise and Heart Failure. *Circulation*, **107**, 1210.

Pollock, M.L., Franklin, B.A., Balady, G.D. & Chaitman, B.L. (2000). Resistance exercise in individuals with and without cardiovascular disease. *Circulation*, **101**, 828.

Rosen, S.E., Borer, J.S. & Hochreiter, C. (1994). Natural history of the asymptomatic patient with severe mitral regurgitation. *American Journal of Cardiology.* **74**, 374–80.

Scottish Intercollegiate Guidelines Network (SIGN) (2001). *Diagnosis and Treatment of Heart Failure Due to Left Ventricular Systolic Dysfunction*. Edinburgh.

Scottish Intercollegiate Guidelines Network (SIGN) (2002). *Cardiac Rehabilitation. A national clinical guideline*. Edinburgh.

Squires, R.W. (1998). *Exercise prescription for the high-risk cardiac patient. Human Kinetics*, Champaign.

Stevenson, L.W., Brunken, R.C. & Belil, D. (1990). Afterload reduction with vasodilators and diuretics decreases metal regurgition during upright exercise in advanced heart failure. *Journal of American College of Cardiology*, **15**, 174–80.

The Acute Infarction Ramipril Efficacy (AIRE) Study Investigators (1993). Effect of ramipril on mortality and morbidity of survivors of acute myocardial infarction with clinical evidence of heart failure. *Lancet,* **342**, 821–8.

Tyni-Lenne, R., Dencker, K., Gordon, A. & Sylven, C. (2001). Comprehensive local muscle training increases aerobic working capacity and quality of life and decreases neurohormonal activation in patients with chronic heart failure. *European Journal of Heart Failure*, **3** (1), 47–52.

Watson, R.D.S., Gibbs, C.R. & Lip, G.Y.H. (2000). ABC of heart failure. Clinical features and complications. *British Medical Journal.* **320**, 236–9.

Bibliography

Aquilani, R., Opasich, C., Dossena, M. & Indarola, P. (2005). Increased skeletal muscle amino acid release with light exercise in deconditioned patients with heart failure. *Journal of American College of Cardiology.* **45**, 158–60.

Michelle Kerr

Meyer, K., Samek, L. & Schwaibold, M. (1996). Physical responses to different modes of interval exercise in patients with chronic heart failure – application to exercise training. *European Heart Journal,* 17, 1040–7.

Middlekauf, H.R., Nitzsche, E.U. & Hamilton, M.A. (2000). Exaggerated renal vasoconstriction during exercise in heart failure patients. *Circulation,* 101, 784.

Chapter 10

Improved symptom control in palliative care for heart failure[1]

Barbara Flowers

Although prognosis for those with heart failure is difficult to predict, it is generally accepted that when severe there is a one year survival rate of less than 50 per cent. For those with mild to moderate heart failure this percentage increases to 20 to 30 per cent (Squire 2005).

As the condition advances the focus for management needs to change to address unresolved symptoms and complex end of life issues alongside active care. Historically the health services have been geared towards dealing with acute episodes of failure, but over the last few years the increasing priority of sensitive and responsive palliative care has become a matter of public policy. In 2000 the National Service Framework for Coronary Heart Disease (DoH 2000) stated that services should: 'help people with unresponsive heart failure and other malignant presentations of coronary heart disease receive appropriate palliative care and support'. Cardiac, renal and respiratory symptoms are complicated often by co-morbidities and complex drug regimes, and patients are often elderly. Symptom control at the advanced stages of heart failure must be considered along with appropriate continued active treatment.

It is clear that nurses can exercise their role in symptom control with medication, communication and understanding to support people in the advanced stages and near the end of life.

The issues around the need for a focus on the care for those at the advanced stages of heart failure have recently been addressed on a national and local level. There are symptom control guidelines (Working party of the Merseyside and

Cheshire specialist palliative care and cardiac clinical networks) and the Coronary Heart Disease Collaborative has produced a document addressing co-ordination of care, practical guidance and offering information around services available and communication issues. In many areas the palliative care services have worked alongside the cardiology teams to improve care – the Specialist Palliative Care Team can offer input and advice, and GPs and consultants can refer to the palliative medicine consultant for an opinion, taking advantage of their experience caring for the dying. The multi-disciplinary team including pharmacists, physiotherapists, occupational therapists and counsellors can all impact on an improved uptake. Recognition that the patient has entered the dying phase has led to more uptake of social benefits such as DS 1500 where the patient is not expected to survive more than six months, and the disability allowance where the patient is under 65 years old.

Although prognostic indicators are available it is hard to be accurate, and the disease process is not a steady decline. Markers of a poor prognosis include the following: degree of functional limitation, profound weakness, low sodium, worsening renal function, increased breathlessness, symptomatic low blood pressure, arrhythmias, increased episodes of acute left ventricular failure and increased episodes of decompensation leading to fluid overload.

These signs may signal the opportunity for health professionals to discuss disease progression with patients and those close to them and to help them understand there may be limited time left to them. This can be difficult, as Ward (2002) identified in acknowledging inadequate communication with heart failure patients. Rogers (2000) found that lack of knowledge about the condition and prognosis can lead to anxiety and depression. Guidance in communication can be found in the Coronary Heart Disease Collaborative: Supportive and palliative care for advanced heart failure (Modernisation Agency 2004).

The following contains some practical suggestions around symptom control aimed at those caring for people at the end stages of heart failure. For further information especially drug information see the Symptom Control Guidelines for patients with end stage heart failure.

Improved symptom control in palliative care

Patients suffer varying degrees of symptoms, and for many their main complaint is complete lack of energy. Symptoms to be aware of include the following: dyspnoea, orthopnoea, paroxysmal nocturnal dyspnoea (PND), sleep disordered breathing, fatigue, weakness, immobility, daytime sleepiness, fluid imbalance – dehydration, fluid overload, symptomatic low blood pressure – light-headedness, confusion, cognitive impairment, agitation, low mood, anxiety, depression, pain, discomfort, constipation, dysuria, anorexia, cardiac cachexia, poor response to medication changes, urinary and/or faecal incontinence, poor tissue viability and pruritus.

Symptom management

Symptom management

Research has shown that pain, dyspnoea and mental disturbance are frequently reported at the end stages of heart failure (McCarthy *et al.* 1996). It is important to remember that symptoms can always be due to co-morbid conditions, or may be as a result of medication. Assessment of these and other symptoms can provide clues as to what may help.

Breathlessness

Assessment of breathlessness can include the following questions alongside clinical examination:

When are you short of breath – how often, what brings it on, what helps? If GTN spray or other nitrates help then the breathlessness is probably ischaemic. If inhalers or nebulisers help then the cause is probably chronic obstructive pulmonary disease (COPD)/asthma. If position or rest helps then it is probably due to heart failure. It is necessary to know if there is breathlessness at rest or on exertion. How far can you walk, how do you manage stairs, how long does it take to recover? Do you have a cough, is it productive or dry, do you expectorate? What is the phlegm like – if it is mucoid what is its colour – if discoloured then possible infection or COPD, a specimen will identify cause of infection and indicate an antibiotic if appropriate. If sputum is frothy or bubbly, and possibly pink tinged then it is probably fluid congestion from heart failure. This should respond to adjustment or increase in diuretics – adding a thiazide to loop diuretics if full doses are already in place. This can be adjusted according to response, try alternate days initially, and increase or reduce as needed. Changing time of dose may help – if breathlessness is mainly at night the diuretic may be needed later in the day – avoiding sleep disturbance is usually the rationale for morning diuretics but this needs to be balanced with disturbed sleep through dyspnoea. Nitrates also improve breathlessness due to heart failure as vasodilators; aim for doses that should not impact too much on low blood pressure.

If more than two pillows are used the cause may be orthopnoea. If there are episodes of waking up suddenly short of breath this could be paroxysmal nocturnal dyspnoea, both these would respond to diuretics.

Excess fluid on the lungs can be acute or insidious. Acute situations – paroxysmal nocturnal dyspnoea (PND) may be described by the sufferer using the following expressions: 'woken up suddenly', 'fighting for breath', 'had to sit up', 'slept in the chair', 'can't go to bed', 'felt panicky', 'awful feeling'. Sitting up can relieve this, with legs over the side of the bed (to relieve fluid pressure) and leaning on a table or window ledge with elbows out. This can happen several times a night, often stage IV on the NYHA scale sufferers will not sleep in a bed, but stay on a recliner or armchair. If this is not improved by these actions then pulmonary oedema can follow – requiring hospital admission and intravenous frusemide, diamorphine, maxolon and possibly nitrates. This may be described by patients as feeling as if they are drowning, causing real fear and panic. Reassurance should be given that on dialling 999 help is very near, and relief can be administered quickly.

The term sleep disordered breathing (SDB) describes episodes of repeatedly waking up gasping for breath. It has been found to be common in those with heart failure – affecting 51 to 68 per cent of patients (Vazir et al. 2005, Jahaveri et al. 1998, Sin et al. 1999). This may be the cause of what patients describe as 'panic attacks', and can disturb sleep over a long period of time. The psychological and physical effects of this impact on quality of life, patients will describe wakening suddenly, or not managing to get completely to sleep, jerking awake with feelings of breathlessness, heart racing and possible panic. Possible treatment may include assessment for Continuous Positive Airway Pressure (CPAP).

Oxygen may help in end stage heart failure especially if there are co-morbidities such as COPD, although assessment with saturation measurements may not indicate its use. The doctor will determine the required dose. Nasal cannulae are more comfortable and allow talking and eating while using oxygen, and two cylinders will avoid the risk of running out. The hazards should be explained to ensure safety.

The position of the patient may help with respiration but it might also indicate that the patient's condition is getting worse. Sitting upright in a chair may be more comfortable for the patient, lying down becomes difficult as the relaxation of the patient allows abdominal contents to inhibit the free movement of the diaphragm. Raising oedematous limbs can also cause fluid to drain back into the central circulation with the risk of congestion to the lungs.

Opiates are used in the mainstream treatment of acute, treatable heart failure. But they can also be used in end stage heart failure, not primarily for their analgesic properties but rather in reducing anxiety, reducing breathlessness and through their effect on haemodynamics (Davies & Curtis 2000). Many writers including Ward (2002) have made the point that 'there is no practical reason why the regular use of morphine should not be considered as routine for the treatment of the dyspnoea of chronic heart failure'. Others have gone further and argued that 'with the collaboration of patient, family and home health services, morphine therapy may prevent hospitalisation when other therapeutic options have been exhausted' (Fischer 1998). Indeed Doyle (1998) pointed out that the after-load reducing action of morphine improves cardiac function.

Simple measures such as relaxation and breathing techniques, a cool room and a fan can help relieve breathlessness, and others can help in this. Cough can be eased with oromorph at the end stages of heart failure if other measures such as linctus or changing Angiotensin Converting Enzyme inhibitors to Angiotensin Receptor Blockers have not helped.

Fatigue

Fatigue can be exacerbated by several factors – anaemia, poor sleep patterns, low blood pressure, medication, thyroid inefficiency or inadequate nutrition. Full assessment may identify causes that can be addressed. Adjusting medication or doses of medication may help, for example lowering the dose of beta-blockers or separating out the timing of medication. Fatigue can be one of the first symptoms that a patient may complain of in developing heart failure, but it is likely to become much worse as the patient enters the terminal phase of the disease. It is well that patients and family are prepared for this, as changes in family roles may need adapting to. Again simple measures can make a difference e.g. the loan of a wheelchair or stair lift, bringing the bed downstairs. Occupational therapy assessment can help with practical aids.

The balance between worsening renal function, symptom control and low blood pressure can be aided by assessment and adjustment of medication to control symptoms such as diuretics, nitrates and those to prevent deterioration in long-term heart function, statins or beta-blockers. This assessment can include the frequency of blood tests for kidney function, which we know may deteriorate. Is it necessary to keep such an accurate picture of blood chemistry, can all blood tests be done at one time to avoid frequent needles? If an increase in diuretics is needed to reduce oedema or to treat pulmonary congestion then it may help to reduce or temporarily withdraw ACE inhibitors to protect compromised blood pressure or kidney function. There is always the risk of dehydration especially with large doses of diuretics, and this can also reduce blood pressure further. Signs of dehydration can be detected without blood tests, monitoring fluid intake and output without compromising the dignity of the patient can indicate a stable fluid balance.

Low mood, anxiety and depression

These mood states are widely reported among heart failure patients. They may be the response of perfectly rational people to a bleak and uncertain future. Spiritual care for believers may have a role to play here, for others the simple solidarity of friends family and neighbours may offer some relief, as will confidence in the team caring for them.

There are options with drug therapy. The selective serotonin reuptake inhibitors are useful and well tolerated, and have the advantage of being less cardio toxic than tricyclic antidepressants with less of a tendency to cause sudden death (Simon &

Gibbs 2001). The benefit at end stage is not clear. Clinical psychologists have a role to play here if referral is possible. Cognitive impairment can be a part of long-term poor perfusion, unusual confusion may be as a result of hypoxia and oxygen therapy may be of benefit. For more information on drug treatment of anxiety and agitation at end stage see the symptom control guidelines.

Sleep disorders

Full assessment of the cause of sleeplessness may show that treating other symptoms can help – dyspnoea, discomfort, fear, or practical issues such as nocturia. Often dozing during the daytime means quality sleep at night is difficult. See the Guidelines for medication considerations.

Loss of appetite, poor nutritional status

Fluid congestion can cause the feeling of being bloated and full. This can be present even with no peripheral oedema, and often the arms and legs can be thin towards the end stages of heart failure as muscle wasting advances. A typical picture can be of boney neck, shoulders and upper arms, and distended abdomen, and there may be a yellow tinge due to liver congestion. Ascites, congestion and constipation can all reduce appetite, and absorption of any nutrition or medication can be compromised. The Scottish Intercollegiate Guidelines Network (SIGN) (1999) identified cachexia as a frequent complication of advanced heart failure, and that this can exacerbate exercise intolerance and reduce muscle mass. Small amounts of food offered regularly supplemented by nutritious drinks should be encouraged. High-energy foods can be offered, as often cholesterol levels may be low at this stage of the condition. This may be a challenge as the advice is usually a low fat diet with heart complaints. This may be an opportunity to reassess the need for statin medication. Other essential medication may be administered in alternative forms to ensure absorption as the gastrointestinal tract may eventually be unreliable – subcutaneous, intravenous – although this may necessitate hospital inpatient stays – rectal, transdermal, buccal or sublingual. It is generally accepted that avoiding salt is essential at all stages of heart failure – even if serum sodium is low. This may be due to dilution rather than low salt intake, and raising intake will cause an increase in fluid retention.

Elimination

At the end stages of any condition constipation can cause severe discomfort. With heart failure this is a risk for several reasons – the usual advice to avoid constipation is impractical. An increase in fluid intake may not be advisable or possible, encouragement to increase activity unrealistic due to fatigue and a high fibre diet unpalatable and too bulky. The energy to push or strain at stool may be absent. Motility of the large bowel can be compromised due to congestion and poor perfusion. Assessment of normal bowel habits can indicate the need for aperients. These should be started early, and a pattern established and maintained, especially if morphine medication is used.

Urinary frequency and continence problems

Frequency can be a problem at all stages of heart failure. Nocturia can be described as common. Diuretic use makes the availability of toilets a constant priority and it may be the practical problems of getting to the toilet or lack of energy that needs to be addressed. This may be a temptation for sufferers to miss doses of diuretics or reduce fluid intake, and can contribute to low mood. In the later stages consider the use of urinary catheters, conveens and other continence aids, with the priority of comfort, dignity and cleanliness.

Oedema

Oedema can be the source of considerable discomfort to a dying patient. The earlier a build up of fluid is detected the sooner changes in diuretic doses can control it, monitoring of daily weight is still a priority where practical. It is not always detected just in the ankles or lower limbs, and it is worth remembering that loss of weight through reduced muscle mass can mask an increase in weight in fluid. Thiazides and aldosterone antagonists with constant monitoring of effect can augment loop diuretics in adjusted doses according to response. This may involve daily or alternate day assessment, and if used carefully can reduce the need for renal function monitoring. Again the combination of diuretics may reduce the risk of raised or lowered serum potassium levels, and limited use of thiazides can help to avoid sodium depletion. Quinine can be given for cramps.

There may be a place for referral to the lymphoedema nurse. In all cases skin may become very friable and at risk of cellulitis and ulcers. Often at very end stage oedema is not a problem, and the aim is a balance between aggressive treatment of fluid overload and comfort measures.

Pain

Pain is reported as a common symptom at the end stages of heart failure, but its cause can be difficult to identify. A full assessment will give clues as to what may trigger the pain, what helps to relieve it. As many patients are elderly and may have co-morbidities it may not necessarily be due to the heart failure. Osteo or rheumatoid arthritis is common, and the neurological pain of diabetes. Ischaemic pain can be treated with nitrates; anti-inflammatory drugs are best avoided except for very short-term use when nothing else helps. The use of the World Health Organisation (1990) pain scale is appropriate, although originally designed for use in the context of cancer it can be applied in cardiology. Where codeine based medication and opiates are used aperients are essential. Basic comfort measures and relaxation will help.

Skin

Skin care is an issue at the end stage of any condition as immobility increases. In heart failure this is also compromised by reduced nutrition, the possibility of dehydration, repeated oedema and pruritus. Pressure relieving mattresses and cushions are essential, and electric beds with the facility to raise the head or lower the legs via remote control where available. The legs and sacrum are at particular risk of breaking down. Fluid can seep from the lower limbs when leg oedema is excessive, dressings may not help as they become wet very quickly. It may be more comfortable to leave the legs exposed, resting on soft towels while seepage is evident. Pruritus may have many causes, liver congestion and poor kidney function can contribute and are difficult to address. It may be a side effect of medication, but whatever the cause it can be severe and distressing. Regular prescriptions of antihistamines can help, and the application of creams such as aqueous cream with 0.5 per cent menthol.

In conclusion full individual assessment involving each patient is essential to identify physical, psychological and spiritual needs. End stage care for those with heart failure has a long way to go, but basic nursing care applied appropriately plus experience and knowledge through the existing palliative care services helps to move towards the aims of the National Service Framework. There remain problems, including defining end stage and improving communication skills, but increasing interest, raised awareness and ongoing research is continually adding to the base of evidence.

Note

1. An earlier treatment of this subject was published in March 2003 in the *Nursing Times*, 99 (11) 30–32, and permission to adapt this chapter has been granted by that publisher..

References

Davies, N. & Curtis, M. (2000). Providing palliative care in end-stage heart failure. *Professional Nurse*, 15, 389–92.

Doyle, D., Hanks, G. & MacDonald, N. (1998). *Oxford Textbook of Palliative Medicine*, 2nd edn. 598.

Fischer, M.D. (1998). Chronic heart failure and morphine treatment. Letters to the Editor. *Mayo Clinic Proceedings*, 73, 194–5.

Gibbs, L.M., Addington-Hall, J. & Gibbs, J.S. (1998). Dying from heart failure: lessons from palliative care. *British Medical Journal*, 317, 961–2.

Javaheri, S., Parker, T., Liming J., Corbett, B.S., Nishiyama, H., Wexler, L. & Roselle, G.A. (1998). Sleep apnoea in 81 ambulatory male patients with stable heart failure: Types and their prevalences, consequences, and presentations. *Circulation*, 97, 2154–9

Levenson, J., McCarthy, E., Lynn J., Davies, R.B. & Phillipps, R.S. (2000). The last six months of life for patients with congestive heart failure. *Journal of the American Geriatric Society*, 48 (5 Suppl.), 101–9.

Pitt, B., Zannad, F., Remme, W.J., Cody, R., Castaigne, A., Perez, A., Palensky, J. & Wittes, J. (1999). The effect of spironalactone on morbidity and mortality in patients with severe heart failure. Randomised aldactone evaluation study investigators. *The New England Journal of Medicine*, 341 (10), 709–17.

Rogers, A., Addington-Hall, J., Abery A.J., McCoy, A.S., Bulpitt, C., Coats, A.J. & Gibbs, J.S. (2000). Knowledge and communication difficulties for patients with chronic heart failure: qualitative study. *British Medical Journal*, 321 (7261), 605–7.

Scottish Intercollegiate Guidelines Network (SIGN) (1999). Sign Secretariat, Royal College of Physicians. Edinburgh.

Simon, J. & Gibbs, R. (2001). Heart disease, in Addington-Hall, J. & Higginson I. (eds). *Palliative care for non-cancer patients*. Oxford: Oxford University Press.

Sin, D.D., Fitzgerald, F., Parker, J., Newton, G., Floras, J.S. & Bradley, T.D. (1999). Risk factors for central and obstructive sleep apnoea in 450 men and women with congestive heart failure. *American Journal Respiratory Critical Care Medicine*, 160, 1101–6.

Vazir, A., Morrell, M., Simonds, A. & McIntyre, H. (2005). Sleep-disordered breathing and heart failure: an opportunity missed? *British Journal of Cardiology*, 12, 219–23.

Ward, C. (2002). The need for palliative care in the management of heart failure. *Heart*, 87, 294–8.

Barbara Flowers

World Health Organisation (1990). *Pain relief and palliative care*. Technical Report Series 804. Geneva: WHO.

Bibliography

Cleland J., Dargie H. & Ford L. (1987). Mortality in heart failure: clinical variables of prognostic value. *British Heart Journal*, **58**, 572–82.

Department of Health (2000). *National Service Framework for Coronary Heart Disease. Modern standards and service models*. London: The Stationery Office.

Department of Health (2004). NHS Modernisation Agency – Coronary Heart Disease *Collaborative. supportive and palliative care for advanced heart failure*. London: The Stationery Office.

McCarthy, M., Lay, M. & Addington-Hall, J. (1996). Dying from heart disease. Journal of the Royal College of Physicians of London, **30** (4), 325-8.

McCarthy, M., Addington-Hall, J. & Lay M. (1997). Communication and choice in dying from heart disease. *Journal of the Royal Society of Medicine*, **90** (3), 128–31.

Millar, B. (1998). Palliative care for people with non-malignant diseases. *Nursing Times*, **94** (48), 52–3.

O'Brien, T., Welsh, J. & Dunn, F. (1998). ABC of palliative care: Non-malignant conditions. *British Medical Journal,* **316**, 286–9.

Trouce, J. & Gould, D. (1997). *Clinical pharmacology for nurses* (15th ed.), Edinburgh: Churchill Livingstone.

Weatherall, D. J., Ledingham, J.G. & Warrell, D.A. (1996). *Oxford Textbook of Medicine* (3rd edn.). Oxford: Oxford University Press.

Chapter 11

Improving palliative care service provision for patients with heart failure[1]

Clare Lewis

More evidence now suggests that heart failure is increasing in incidence and has an increasing mortality (DoH 2000b, SHAPE Investigators 2003). Heart failure is an area of major concern for health service planners and it is predicted to rise by approximately 70 per cent by the year 2015, translating into 1.5 million new cases (SHAPE Investigators 2003). This is a condition of high mortality. It is estimated in the UK that 16 per cent of patients will die within the first month after diagnosis and 40 per cent of patients will be dead at the end of year one (British Heart Foundation 2005).

In an attempt to improve quality of life and survival rates, the Government published the National Service Framework (NSF) (DoH 2000b) for Coronary Heart Disease and more recently the National Institute for Clinical Excellence (NICE) heart failure guidelines (NICE 2003). The primary aims of these documents were to confirm the diagnosis of heart failure, commence appropriate pharmacological measures, slow progression of the disease and thereby reduce hospital admissions and improve life expectancy. In addition to medication regimes, techniques such as Cardiac Resynchronisation Therapy (CRT) and Automatic Internal Cardiac Defibrillators (AICD) have demonstrated improvements in mortality rates and reduction in hospital admissions (Cleland *et al.* 2001, Bristow *et al.* 2004). Also, with management of heart failure by specialist nurses, patients have demonstrated overall greater awareness of their illness, have increased their compliance and have reported an improved quality of life (Blue *et al.* 1999, Palmer *et al.* 2003).

However, although these public policy developments have raised the standard of what patients can expect in the way of cardiology services, the questions of what to do when the patient enters the terminal stage of their illness is not addressed in any satisfying way either by the NSF or in the NICE guidelines. That said, the fact that these questions are raised at all is in itself an advance on previous years. This represents some recognition at last of the enormity of the problems facing the patient who must face cancer type life expectancy with support from health care services which have hitherto been poorly equipped to respond (McCarthy *et al.* 1996, 1997, Addington-Hall 1998, Doyle 1998, Ward 2002, Davidson *et al.* 2004, Segal *et al.* 2005).

Palliative care in heart failure

Palliative care

With the increasing incidence of heart failure managing these patients appropriately is more than ever at the forefront of health care management, especially with the introduction of the NSF for the management of long-term conditions (DoH 2005a) which recognises the needs of those living with a chronic illness. Although not specific to heart failure the framework can be adapted to any chronic disease when addressing the care of patient and family holistically. Of course the publication of this document is a good start. But it is just a start, and services which address the needs of dying patients, a difficult and heterogeneous group, are still frequently under-developed.

There is nothing new in the recognition that heart failure patients have special and difficult to meet needs. Over forty years ago investigators studied the suffering of patients with heart failure and observed anxiety and depression to complicate the physical burden of heart failure (Hinton 1963). It is not as though the pain of heart failure is only physical. Study after study have demonstrated that the suffering of heart failure patients is all encompassing and extends way beyond the person with pump failure (Addington-Hall 1998, Doyle 1998, Field & Addington-Hall 1999, Koenig 1998, Segal *et al.* 2005). In a study conducted by Koenig (1998) it was determined that 36 per cent of patients with heart failure had major depression. It should be emphasised that this does not mean that they were excessively sad, rather that they had severe, treatable, mental dysfunction. It is not clear however that these patients are actually treated.

The studies of patients' histories who die from heart failure make grim and unrewarding reading. Addington-Hall and McCarthy's 1990 study set the tone for many of these studies and illuminated the final months of a patient's life, as recalled by their carers. Their story was one of distress and suffering with little or no relief. It was typically a story which compared to the worst of patients with cancer but with little of the specialised support available to patients with the latter condition. Typical symptoms varied, including breathlessness, pain, low mood, sleeplessness, urinary and faecal incontinence, loss of appetite, mental confusion, nausea and vomiting.

Of course carers' recollections might be subject to all sorts of accuracy-distorting influences but there have been few studies which have contradicted Addington-Hall and McCarthy's findings. Quite the reverse, although more research would sharpen the picture, the trend in all the current research paints a depressingly consistent tableau (Lynn *et al.* 1997, Addington-Hall 1998, Doyle 1998, Juenger *et al.* 2002, Murray *et al.* 2002, Ward 2002, Lewis & Stephens 2005). A poor quality, badly supported life comes across again and again.

As death becomes imminent, things hardly improve. A proportion of patients (15 per cent) have been demonstrated to undergo resuscitation attempts even up to the last three days before dying (Lynne *et al.* 1997). A further 40 per cent underwent aggressive treatment up to and including mechanical ventilation, even though 48 per cent said that they would prefer comfort measures to help them with their uncontrolled dyspnoea (66 per cent) or their 'severe pain' (45 per cent). This is very depressing if it is representative.

Medical prescription of these aggressive techniques is clearly hard to defend where the patient is so close to death. However it can be notoriously difficult to pin point the moment that heart failure enters its end stage (Lynn *et al.* 1997). It has been pointed out again and again that death from heart failure is not as 'linear' as many other malignant conditions (Ward 2002 and Ellershaw & Ward 2003). Anybody who has looked after a patient with heart failure will be aware of occasions when a patient apparently hours from dying has made a last minute 'Lazarus' style recovery. It is this last fact that makes the decision to desist in active treatment so difficult and why a gap has opened between the patient with, say, fulminant cancer and the patient with heart failure. Here again, the figures speak for themselves. Though arguably most people with heart failure would prefer to die at home, a full 58 per cent have been shown to die in hospital. Only 27 per cent died at home, with access to hospice care reserved for the lucky 3 per cent (Lynn *et al.* 1997). In spite of the rhetoric which trumpets the superiority of hospice care over hospital care when the patient is dying (Wallston *et al.* 1998), the reality is that hospice places will be beyond the reach of all but a tiny minority of heart failure patients (Doyle 1998, Zambroski 2004).

Direct comparisons of the fates of heart failure and lung cancer victims make equally sobering reading. While nobody would be inclined to describe a lung cancer victim as lucky exactly, nevertheless heart failure patients can seem disadvantaged in comparison. Take the issue of information for instance. Some studies have compared the insight into their condition which heart failure patients have unfavourably with that of cancer patients (Murray *et al.* 2002). As if the physical discomfort of this condition were not enough, this study pointed to the extra suffering which uncertainty about one's fate imposed on victims of heart failure. Both patient and carer in this study did not feel a part of decisions about plans of care, and carers expressed that they felt exhausted and isolated.

This inequity has not escaped health service planners. The Cancer Plan (DoH 2000a) recognised the need for palliative care to extend beyond cancer and to take account of the needs of the patient rather than the needs of the disease process. However service provision needs to develop to match this public policy commitment. There is some evidence that this is starting to happen with teams of nurses beginning to incorporate the expertise of HF specialist nurses (Segal *et al.* 2005).

Barriers to provision

Barriers to the provision of palliative care services in heart failure

Providing palliative care in heart failure is hampered by lack of insight by health professionals who focus on invasive aggressive treatments which increase survival rather than quality of life for patient and family (Doyle *et al.* 1993, Addington-Hall & McCarthy 1995, Linden 1995, Segal *et al.* 2005, Lewis & Stephens 2005).

Though the patient and the family may welcome and appreciate the care offered, Specialist Practitioner in Palliative Care (SPPC) is often introduced at too late a stage for its benefit to be maximised. Of course the difficulty in pinpointing the end stage of the condition does not help, with acute and chronic episodes exchanging places periodically (Doyle 1998).

The very name of palliative care is perhaps less than completely helpful. 'Palliative care' tends to be associated with cancer in the public's, the patient's and carers' minds. The public especially require education here. The SHAPE Investigators (2003) examined the knowledge base of nearly 8,000 people in nine countries. They discovered that a full 70 per cent did not consider heart failure a serious condition, while 65 per cent thought that survival was longer for people with heart failure than for people with cancer. As the prevalence of heart failure is expected to rise, publicity relating to this condition will increase and awareness may actually encourage patients and family to ask questions about the illness and the treatment options. Not before time.

Communication issues

Communication, as Albert *et al.* (2002) highlights is overall the most important aspect of patient care and if inadequate can result in sub-optimal provision. Poor communication between health professionals and patients and carers is a recognised fact in the management of HF (Gibbs *et al.* 1998, Murray *et al.* 2002, Edmonds *et al.* 2005). Poor communication can result in misinformation about treatment options and result in lack of insight and awareness about diagnosis and life expectancy (Gibbs *et al.* 1998, Murray *et al.* 2002). Problems resulting from poor communication in HF have been identified by Rogers *et al.* (2000). Within this study patients reported that they felt they had limited opportunities to raise questions about their condition. While some patients felt that they respected the doctors' knowledge, many also said that the doctor was reluctant to give too much information or felt the doctor presumed they did not have the ability to understand. These misconceptions and misunderstandings can impinge on developing plans of care. They can lead to each side in the care equation not really knowing what is needed or required from the other.

Communication can be affected by time restrictions, pressures of workload and an inability to facilitate open communication. This can lead to poorly co-ordinated services. (Fuat *et al.* 2003). In order to address this problem a multi-disciplinary team approach is of paramount importance in treating patient and family holistically.

Hospice care

Hospice care

The hospice movement has an important part in managing this group of individuals and their carers whether they be inpatients or outpatients. Evidence from Lynn *et al.* (1997) demonstrated that only 3 per cent of patients with heart failure were offered the option of a hospice place. Thorns and Gibbs (2001) undertook a retrospective, UK based study, investigating service demand of heart failure patients. Their study focused on one hospice between the years 1994 and 1999. Alarmingly, out of 9920 referrals only 27 were for heart failure and from these a total of only 19 were accepted. Given the numbers of people with heart failure, this seems an alarmingly low order of provision.

A study by Zambroski (2004) investigated this sparse uptake of services. The study highlighted diminutive awareness by health professionals of the role of the hospice and services offered. Of course it could also be that hospices themselves are not fully inclined to advertise their services in case they are swamped by non–cancer terminally ill patients who squeeze out their traditional clientele. As hospices depend on charitable funding there have been concerns that cancer charities may relinquish funds if they divert their services to heart failure patients. Furthermore, if beds are occupied by those with heart failure there is concern that cancer patients may be turned away (Doyle 1998).

Lack of confidence and skills to provide care for heart failure patients within a hospice is also a concern of hospice workers. To overcome this problem Doyle (1998) suggests close working links with the health professionals who referred the patient. To bolster the confidence of hospice workers, specialist personnel in the cardiac services could repay the assistance given by the hospice staff by sharing their skills. Consultant cardiologists, specialist nurses, nutritionists, physiotherapists and pharmacists could all co-operate in the delivery of care, and in demystifying each other's contribution to terminal care.

Palliative care in the community

Palliative care in the community

Although there is a depressing tendency for people with heart failure to die in hospital, the majority of their care up to the end will be managed in the community. What is more, the pressure on the NHS to keep them in the community will increase as the population ages and the secondary services struggle to cope with increasing numbers (DOH 2005a). Yet the care of patients with chronic conditions is one where the health-care planners and the users of services have a common interest. It is accepted that high quality care can be delivered to patients' homes and their (complex) needs met. This will be welcome news to many elderly people who would prefer to have those services at home.

Of course, nothing is that simple. Some serious questions hang over this strategy. Difficulties with delivering care in this way have been examined by Fuat *et al.* in 2003. They discovered that general practitioners lacked confidence in the management of heart failure patients. Further, they felt that they did not have time to incorporate heavily time consuming palliative care techniques into their already overstretched diaries. Little confidence was expressed in this study in the degree of support which would be forthcoming from, say, the cardiologist. This is a telling point as the complex medication patterns of people in heart failure can require some detailed technical opinion.

Perhaps the difficulties here can mask opportunities. Perhaps it is about time that specialist palliative services ought to develop their knowledge of cardiac problems. And maybe cardiac services ought to familiarise themselves with palliative care techniques. Further, maybe the vehicle for this expansion in expertise is close co-operation between teams in the community.

This is the type of joined up approach that report after report has advocated.

Lack of understanding about the Specialist Practitioner in Palliative Care and its role in managing heart failure is a great issue (Addington-Hall 1998, Doyle 1998). In spite of this Doyle (1998) and Ellershaw and Ward (2003) recognise that palliative care techniques are neither secret nor mysterious and can be employed by anyone in health and social care involved in managing these patients and their families.

The palliative care approach

The palliative care approach

Palliation is not only about medication and alleviating physical symptoms. It is about ensuring the patients' needs and those of their families are recognised and addressed with appropriate service provision in place. Ellershaw and Ward (2003) and Hauptman and Havranek (2005) emphasise those aspects of palliative care which concern open communication and optimising symptoms. They affirm the central place of the patient and family in decision-making and psychosocial care. No one person will have the most expertise in all fields. One person cannot provide all of this care. Nothing does this as effectively as a team approach.

The main goal in the provision of palliative care in community services is to develop expertise in the whole team, reserving Specialist Practitioner in Palliative Care and Cardiology for a consultative role. Some studies have provided evidence that home based services can promote greater communication, greater awareness of patients' wishes, improved self care management and better collaboration on a multi-professional level (Albert *et al.* 2002).

Naturally, none of this is cheap. To keep people out of hospital new and more acceptable ways of working need to be developed. More resources will be required to support people at home. Equipment, respite care, training for the myriad partners in care will be required, as will the advice and support from hospices and hospitals when things do not go to plan. But the cost of these services is already being borne by an NHS which picks up the costs of inappropriate care and emergency admissions.

Gold standards framework

The Gold Standards Framework (GSF) in community palliative care management was developed in the UK to address issues of lack of co-ordination and sub-optimal service provision for cancer patients in the last 6–12 months of life (Thomas 2002). Although developed for patients with cancer it can be adopted when caring for patients with heart failure. Its aim is transferable in that it ensures patient and family are central to the management and service provision including preferred place of care. Initial reports have suggested that this framework has resulted in fewer problems developing when mainstream services are closed, in better symptom control, more financial support for carers and greater collaboration all around (Thomas 2002).

The framework is not difficult to use and permits a unified and timely update of a patient's condition and the recording of developments in a register. Someone is designated to take the lead in the care of a patient. All of the main participants in care are brought in regularly to review the patient's progress, with specialist services called in when required.

Nominating a person responsible for the co-ordination of the patient's care, in line with GSF recommendations, overcomes one of the most serious problems which face the heart failure patient: the disjointed nature of care delivery (Murray *et al.* 2002). The co-ordinator could be anyone who has regular contact with the patient, their aim being to co-ordinate service provision such as district nurses, GP, heart failure nurses, Specialist Practitioner in Palliative Care nurse, community matron, physiotherapist or occupational therapist or those in social care.

Conclusion

Those with HF and their carers can experience many prolonged symptoms greatly affecting quality of life. Despite research and recommendations within documents such as NSF for heart failure management (DoH 2000b) and NICE Guidelines (2003), service provision and long-term input remain inadequate.

Developing services is affected by the unpredictability of the disease as well as lack of understanding of the principles underpinning palliative care. Poor communication between patient and family and failure to recognise that the patient is moving into the end stages only adds to the difficulties. Funding difficulties and poor public awareness about heart failure also affect development of services. If the public were more aware then they might challenge current service provision. They might demand better treatment options if diagnosed with heart failure.

Greater awareness about the services available for this group of patients needs to be developed. This could be achieved through consultative forums where those in primary care and the acute sector come together and discuss services in their areas.

Government has a large role to play in developing protocols for practice and guidelines for palliative care in heart failure. It could also inject more funding into research projects which look at ways to balance the physical needs of this condition as well as the palliative care needs.

Education and training programmes ought to be developed as part of pre- and post- registration courses both in nursing and medicine as well as training for the voluntary sector and those working within social care.

Further development of frameworks such as the GSF is essential to discourage unco-ordinated care and improved ways of applying the GSF to patients with heart failure need to be considered. As the incidence of heart failure increases services must change and adapt to the needs of this group of individuals and their families. Innovations such as hospices specific to heart failure management and day centres with multi-disciplinary team involvement may be future options.

It is no longer acceptable to ignore the palliative care needs of those with heart failure believing it to be solely the responsibility of the Specialist Practitioner in Palliative Care or by using the unpredictability of the disease as a defence. We must as a multi-disciplinary team provide a holistic service and address inequalities to service provision.

1. An earlier treatment of this subject was published in December 2004 in *Primary Health Care* 14 (10) 24–3 and permission to adapt this chapter has been granted by that publisher.

Improving palliative care service provision

References

Addington-Hall, J. & McCarthy, M. (1990). Regional study of care for the dying. *Palliative Medicine*, 9, 27–35.

Addington-Hall, J. (1998). Palliative care in non-malignant disease. *Palliative Medicine*, 10, 7–10.

Addington-Hall, J. & McCarthy, M. (1995). Regional study for the dying: methods and sample characteristics. *Palliative Medicine,* 9, 27–35.

Albert, N. M., Davis, M. & Young, J. (2002). Improving the care of patients dying of heart failure. *Cleveland Clinical Journal of Medicine*, 69 (4), 321–8.

Blue, L., Lang, E., McMurray, J.J., Davie, A.P., McDonagh, T.A., Murdoch, D.R., Petrie, M.C., Connolly, E., Norrie, J., Round, C.E., Ford, I. & Morrison, C.E. (2001). Randomised controlled trial of specialist nurse intervention in heart failure. *British Medical Journal*, 323 (7315), 715–18.

Bristow, M.R., Saxon, L.A., Boehmer, J., Krueger, S., Kass, D.A., DeMarco, T., Carson, P., DiCarlo, L., DeMets, D., White, B.G., DeVries, D.W. & Feldman, A.M. (2004). For the Comparison of Medical Therapy, Pacing and Defibrillation in Heart Failure (COMPANION) Investigators. Cardiac-resynchronisation therapy with or without an implantable defibrillator in advanced chronic heart failure. *The New England Journal of Medicine*, 350 (21), 2140–50.

British Heart Foundation (2005). British Heart Foundation's Statistics Website. www.heartstats.org/

Cleland, J.G.F., Daubert, J.C., Erdmann, E., Freemantle, N., Gras, D., Kappenberger, L., Klein, W. & Tavazzi, L. (2001). The CARE-HF Study (CArdiac REsynchronization in Heart Failure study): rationale, design and endpoints. *The European Journal of Heart Failure*, 3 (4), 481–9.

Davidson, P. M., Paull, G., Introna, K. & Cockburn, J. (2004). Integrated, collaborative palliative care in heart failure: The St. George heart failure service experience 1999-2002. *The Journal of Cardiovascular Nursing*, 19 (1), 68–76.

Department of Health (2000a). *National Council for Hospice and Specialist Palliative Care Services. Cancer Plan*, London: The Stationery Office.

Department of Health, (2000b). *National Service Framework: Modern Standards and Service Models, Coronary Artery Disease, Chapter Six, Heart Failure*. London: The Stationery Office.

Department of Health (2005b). *Supporting People with Long Term Conditions*. London: The Stationery Office.

Doyle, D. (1998). Palliative care for patients with non-malignant disease. National Council for Hospice and Specialist Palliative Care Services and Scottish Partnership Agency for Palliative and Cancer Care, June 1998, Paper 14.

Clare Lewis

Doyle, D., Hanks, G. W. & Macdonald, N. (eds.) (1993). *Palliative Medicine,* Oxford: Oxford University Press.

Edmonds, P.M., Rogers, A.E., Addington-Hall, J.M., McCoy, A.S.M., Coats, A.J.S. & Gibbs, J.S.R. (2005). Patients' descriptions of breathlessness in heart failure. *International Journal of Cardiology*, 98, 61–6.

Ellershaw, J. & Ward, C. (2003). Care of the dying patient, the last hours or days of life. *British Medical Journal*, 326, 30–4.

Field, D. & Addington-Hall, J. (1999). Extending specialist palliative care to all? *Social Science and Medicine*, 48, 1271–80.

Fuat, A., Hungin, A.P. & Murphy, J. (2003). Barriers to accurate diagnosis and effective management of heart failure in primary care: qualitative study. *British Medical Journal*, 326, 196–200.

Gibbs, L.M.E, Addington-Hall, J. & Gibbs, J.S.R. (1998). Dying from heart failure: Lessons from Palliative Care. *British Medical Journal*, 317, 961–2.

Hauptman, P.J. & Havranek, E.P. (2005). Integrating palliative care into heart failure care. *Archives of Internal Medicine*, 165 (4), 374–8.

Hinton, J, (1963). The physical and mental distress of the dying. Quarterly *Journal of Medicine*, 125, 1–21.

Juenger, J., Schellberg, D., Kraemer, S., Haunsletter, A., Zugck, C., Herzog, W. & Haass, M. (2002). Health related quality of life in patients' with congestive heart failure: comparison with other chronic diseases in relation to functional variables. *Heart*, 87, 235–41.

Koenig, H.G (1998). Depression in hospitalized older patients with chronic heart failure. *General Hospital Psychiatry*, 20 (1), 29–43.

Lewis, C. & Stephens, B. (2005). Improving palliative care provision for patients with heart failure. *British Journal of Nursing*, 14 (10), 563–7.

Linden, B. (1995). Severe Heart Failure: A focus on the quality of care. *Nursing Times*, 91 (33), 38–9.

Lynn, J., Teno, J.M., Phillips, R.S., Wu, A.W., Desbiens, N. & Harrold, J. (1997). Perceptions by family members of the dying experience of older and seriously ill patients. *Annals Internal Medicine*, 126, 97–106.

McCarthy, M., Addington-Hall, J. & Lay, M (1996). Dying from heart disease. *Journal of the Royal College of Physicians of London*, 30 (4), 325–9.

McCarthy, M., Addington-Hall, J. & Lay, M (1997). Communication and choice in dying from heart disease. *Journal of the Royal Society of Medicine*, 90, 128–31.

Murray, S.A., Boyd, K., Kendall, M., Worth, A., Benton, T.F. & Clausen, H. (2002). Dying of lung cancer or cardiac failure: prospective study of patients and their carers in the community. *British Medical Journal*, 325, 919–29.

NICE (2003). *Chronic Heart Failure Management of Chronic Heart Failure in Adults in Primary and Secondary Care.* London: NICE.

Palmer, N.D., Appleton, B. & Rodrigues, E. (2003). Specialist nurse -led intervention in outpatients with congestive heart failure. *Disease Management and Health Outcomes*, 11 (11), 693–8.

Rogers, A.E., Addington-Hall, J., Abery, A.J., McCoy, A.S.M., Bulpitt, C., Coats, A.J.S. & Gibbs, J.S.R. (2000). Knowledge and communication difficulties for patients with chronic heart failure. *British Medical Journal*, 321, 605–7.

Segal, D.I., O'Hanlon, D., Rahman, N., McCarthy, D.J. & Gibbs, J.S.R. (2002). Incorporating palliative care into heart failure management a new model of care. *International Journal of Palliative Nursing*, 11(3), 135–6.

SHAPE Investigators (2003). Shape study shows public unaware of heart failure. *British Journal of Cardiology*, 10 (5), 338.

Thomas, K (2002). *Gold Standards Framework in Community Palliative Care.* Cancer Services Collaborative NHS modernisation agency. London: The Stationery Office.

Thorns, A.R. & Gibbs, L.M (2001). Management of severe heart failure by specialist palliative care. *Heart*, 85 (1), 93.

Wallston, K.A., Burger, C., Smith, R.A. & Baugher, R.J. (1988). Comparing the quality of death for hospice and non hospice cancer patients. *Medical Care*, 26, 177–82.

Ward, C. (2002). The need for palliative care in the management of heart failure. *Heart*, 87, 294–8.

Zambroski, C. (2004). Hospice as an alternative model of care for older patients with end stage heart failure. *Journal of Cardiovascular Nursing,* 19 (1), 76–86.

Bibliography

Department of Health (2000a). *National Council for Hospice and Specialist Palliative Care Services. Cancer Plan*, London: The Stationery Office.

Department of Health (2005b). *Supporting People with Long Term Conditions.* London: The Stationery Office.

Hanratty, B., Hibbert, D., Mair, F., May, C., Ward, C., Capewell, S., Litva, A. & Corcoran, G. (2002). Doctors' perceptions of palliative care for heart failure: a focus group study. *British Medical Journal*, 325, 581–5.

Clare Lewis

Stewart, S.& Blue, L. (2001). *Improving Outcomes in Chronic Heart Failure, a Practical Guide to Specialist Nurse Intervention*. London: BMJ books.

Chapter 12

Assisted dying and heart failure

Linda Gladman

Assisted dying is defined as the intentional taking of a patient's life either by act or omission. It is an act which is supposedly in the person's own interest bringing about a death which is painless and gentle, particularly in respect of those suffering from incurable disease (Biggs 2001, Mak *et al.* 2003).

Definitions of assisted dying involve distinctions between active and passive methods, which are drawn according to the manner in which death is procured and relate closely to the legal understanding of act or omission (Mak *et al.* 2003, Dunstan & Royal 1996, Wal & Dillmann 1994). Active assisted dying is a form of assisted dying where one person offers assistance to bring about a person's death. This may be a physician administering a lethal injection with the intention to kill, or physician assisted suicide whereby a prescription is given to a patient for that patient to bring about his/her own death (Biggs 2001, Mak *et al.* 2003, Otlowski 2000). Withholding or withdrawing life prolonging treatment is classified as passive assisted dying (Garrard & Wilkinson 2005, Biggs 2001).

Active assisted dying is currently accepted in other countries. In the American state of Oregon it was legalised in 1997, the Netherlands in 2002 and Belgium in 2002 (Guedj *et al.* 2005, House of Lords 2005). In Britain the common law position has been extensively reviewed and several attempts have been made to reform the law and legalise Physician Assisted Suicide (PAS) (Biggs 2001, Otlowski 2000, House of Lords 2005). At present the law states that assisted suicide is illegal and any positive attempt to end the patient's life is treated as murder, whatever the motive (Biggs 2001). Currently a bill is being considered which would permit the introduction of PAS to the UK, under carefully controlled circumstances. Supporters and opponents of the bill tend to appeal to different basic moral principles. These emphasise autonomy, the prevention of avoidable suffering, the sanctity of life and respect for dignity (Dunstan & Royal 1996, Campbell 2002, Philipsen *et al.* 2005, Emanuel *et al.* 1998, Ward & Tate 1994).

Throughout the countries where it has been accepted there are varying rules for assisted dying. The proposed bill by Lord Joffe states that a patient must be suffering unbearably from a terminal illness. Terminal illness is defined as inevitably progressive in which the effects cannot be reversed by treatment and which will be likely to result in the patient's death within a few months. Under its terms only competent adults can make a request for assistance to die. The definition of competence will rely on the Mental Capacity Act (Mental Capacity Act 2005). The patient must be informed of the prognosis and all other alternatives to assisted dying, including palliative care, must be explored. All requests must be voluntary; however, there are no stated safeguards to ensure that there are no external influences. If a patient's competence is questioned a psychiatric referral should be made to determine that the patient is not suffering from a psychiatric or psychological disorder causing impaired judgement. It is the physician who has primary responsibility for the care of the patient and treatment who will bear the responsibility for overlooking the request for PAS. Lastly there is a 14 day waiting period to allow sufficient time to undertake competence assessments (House of Lords 2005).

Within the above criteria are some interesting features. The definition of terminal illness is wholly dependent upon the consulting physician. What is unbearable suffering? We may recognise it but can we define it? 'Unbearable suffering' is determined by the patient's ability to be able to competently express it to the consulting physician and is open to subjective interpretation by that physician (Magnusson 2004, House of Lords 2005). Another issue to be raised is the potential for arbitrary distinctions to be made between similar patients and with the same patient at different times. For subjective reasons a physician might feel one way about a certain case but feel another way about a similar case at a different time. Consistency cannot be guaranteed as each individual circumstance will be different, with one influencing factor for example being the physician/patient relationship. So this safeguard cannot be wholly effective (Frey 2005, House of Lords 2005). More importantly, if the judgement of a physician was successfully challenged it might throw into doubt all of his/her previous judgements. Could we possibly confirm competence in any human being who is experiencing the emotional turmoil of a serious illness and who is suffering unbearably? Many would suggest that these factors would undermine someone's ability to reason and make a logical and informed choice to die (Rivett 2002, Allmark 2002). The bill also leaves assessment of the patient's competence to the consulting physician and this consultant may not have any special expertise in such assessments, which may have major implications for vulnerable people. Lastly what is meant by 'inform the patient of prognosis and alternative options'? This is an ambiguous phrase and the bill arguably needs to be more specific with regard to the information that should be given.

There are many foreseeable problems with the proposed bill in relation to heart failure patients. Arguably, if a disease is non-malignant (i.e. non-cancer), it is called a condition not a terminal illness. This is despite the fact that it might be incurable and progressive with unbearable suffering (O'Brien *et al.* 1998). Could heart failure patients be accepted as candidates for PAS despite the fact heart failure is not recognised or referred to as terminal (Cushen 1994, Ellershaw & Ward 2003, Jones 1995, Rogers *et al.* 2000, Taylor & Stott 2002)? The bill also suggests that for a patient to fit the criteria, the progression of the illness cannot be reversible by treatment. Prognostication is a huge problem in heart failure patients and determining when the patient has entered the final stage can be very difficult. As found by Hanratty *et al.* (2002) and many others, predicting the illness trajectory and clinical course is extremely difficult in heart failure patients and because of this uncertainty it can virtually paralyse physicians from deciding that patients have entered the terminal stage (Ward 2002, Anderson *et al.* 2001, National Institute for Clinical Excellence 2003, The SUPPORT principle investigators 1995). However other authors have strongly disagreed with this opinion and have argued that end stage heart failure can be predicted with appropriate guidelines and prognostic models suggesting that it is only a lack of research which has prevented this from occurring (Davidson 2002, Goodlin *et al.* 2004, Ellershaw & Ward 2003). In addition Goodlin *et al.* (2004) state that even accepting the difficulty with prognostication there is little excuse for end of life issues to be avoided. Rather they argue that they need to be discussed at an earlier stage in the illness.

Sadly, over-aggressive, unrealistic and 'heroic' treatment still exists for some heart failure patients who are treated inappropriately right up until the last days of life. This is often because of the uncertainty as to whether a patient will respond to treatment (Cushen 1994, Harlan *et al.* 1998). It is not easy to recognise when patients with heart failure are entering the end stages. Sometimes it is not clear that the patient will survive long enough to alert palliative care services. To go the further distance toward a cool and settled request for PAS might be unrealistic for many patients.

A further problem is the incidence of cognitive impairment in heart failure patients. It is widely acknowledged as a phenomenon and might cause huge doubts about the competence and the capacity of patients to make an informed choice. The causes of cognitive impairment in heart failure remain unclear. Dominant themes in the literature suggest cerebral infarction, cerebral hypofusion, low systolic blood pressure and reduced left ventricular ejection fraction (Bennett & Sauve 2003, Acanfora *et al.* 1996, Ekman *et al.* 2001). Within the bill one of the safeguards is that only competent adults can request PAS.

Cognition refers to mental activities relating to thinking, memory and learning (Riegal *et al.* 2002, Bennett & Sauve 2003). Many heart failure patients experience some form of cognitive dysfunction with a reported 80 per cent of patients with severe heart failure experiencing memory deficits, problems with attention, reaction times and concentration (Almeida & Flicker 2001, Ekman *et al.* 2001, Riegel *et al.* 2002, Staniforth *et al.* 2001, Bennett & Sauve 2003). Further studies have shown that patients with chronic heart failure find it difficult to retain information, so patients may not appreciate the relevance of information provided by clinicians. Their ability to put preplanned questions to clinicians is another observed problem which could affect their eligibility for PAS (Wehby & Brenner 1997, Rogers *et al.* 2000, Antonelli et al. 2003). Zuccala *et al.* (1997) revealed 53 per cent of participants had cognitive dysfunction with the biggest deficit in cognition to be that of complex reasoning. Riegel *et al.* (2002) used four screening tools to assess patients and this study revealed 28.6 per cent of the 42 participants had cognitive impairment. Much more literature reveals similar findings. Cognitive impairment is a common problem (Acanfora 1996, Zuccala *et al.* 2001, Cacciatore 1998).

For example, the study by Zuccala *et al.* (1997) found cognitive dysfunction in 53 per cent of their sample as opposed to the 28.6 per cent found by Riegel *et al.* (2002).

Not only do heart failure patients show signs of cognitive impairment but also depression is common with prevalence in outpatients ranging from 11 per cent to 25 per cent (Turvey et al. 2002, Havranek *et al.* 1999). Higher rates were found in hospitalised patients (Gottlieb *et al.* 2004, Rumsfeld *et al.* 2003). The results from the Vaccarino (2001) study were suggestive that the more severely ill the patient the higher the depressive symptoms. Exacerbation of heart failure symptoms increases depressive symptoms. This would reinforce studies carried out on cognition, maybe suggesting some relationship between depression and cognitive impairment. Additionally, current research further reveals that depression in heart failure is often misdiagnosed and untreated (Guck *et al.* 2003 Rumsfeld *et al.* 2003, Vaccarino 2001, Havranek *et al.* 1999, Skotzko *et al.* 2000, Miller 2002). Many nurses will have the experience of seeing physicians regard depressive symptoms as a normal reaction to the progression of the condition and quite often just focus on treatment management plans for heart failure. Many seem to believe in an overlap in symptoms of depression and heart failure. Both show similar signs such as fatigue, dyspneoa, malaise and limited activity (Jacob & Sebastian 2003, Guck 2003, Artinian *et al.* 2004, Havranek *et al.* 1999, Acanfora *et al.* 1996, Rumsfeld *et al.* 2003, Vaccarino 2001).

None of the above puts heart failure patients in a good position to opt for PAS, for the following reasons. The safeguards as they stand for PAS are so complex that heart failure patients may never be able to qualify for assistance (Magnusson 2004). Competence would be a huge issue in this group of patients. The capacity to make a decision on PAS will be based on the patient's appreciation of the following facts: medical diagnosis, prognosis, and the ability to retain that information and weigh that information up as part of making the decision. Having the ability to communicate his/her decision adequately and to understand the process of being assisted to die and alternatives including palliative care may be a hurdle at which many may fall (Mental Capacity Act 2005, House of Lords 2005).

Extensive literature confirms heart failure patients have a poor understanding of their diagnosis. Prognosis is rarely discussed and because of these reasons palliative care in the past has been difficult to initiate (Sloan 2002, Rogers *et al.* 2000, The *et al.* 2000, Gibbs 1998). Communication with these patients presents enduring difficulties. Defining the moment that the patient enters the dying phase and when to initiate palliative care is hardly any easier (Ellershaw & Ward 2003, Davidson 2002, NICE 2003). If PAS is legalised it could have a positive impact upon communication and treatment. Research into patients' reasoning abilities might be mandated to accommodate the legislation, as would the clear statement of alternatives to suicide (Goodlin *et al.* 2004, NSF 2002).

On the other hand a well voiced concern about the legalisation of assisted dying is that vulnerable people will become victims of the legislation. This proposed bill could produce very different approaches from physician to physician (Mak *et al.* 2003, Magnusson 2004, Vaccarino 2001, Davies 2002). Many are sceptical that PAS will give patients more autonomy. They fear that it may increase the authority of doctors over life and death. Some go as far as to question physicians' competence to make morally correct decisions (Sheldon 2004, Mak *et al.* 2003). Concepts like unbearable suffering, terminal illness, depression and competence could be manipulated according to the values of the doctors concerned, or simply ignored (Magnusson 2004). From an opponent's perspective on PAS, one could argue legalised voluntary PAS may lead to involuntary assisted dying because of an untreated or undiagnosed psychological disorder. Depression levels have been shown to fluctuate throughout the course of the illness (Vaccarino 2001). These findings are consistent with those of Friedman *et al.* (2001) who studied 170 patients with heart failure and found 30 per cent of the sample (n = 52) had scores indicative of clinical depression. Interestingly this study showed a decrease in depressive symptoms two weeks following discharge. This in itself is a cause for concern as a patient's thoughts upon the bearability of the condition will vary throughout the course of the illness. Assisted dying, however, is irreversible. Moreover, one could also ponder as to whether the above statistics do not under-represent the prevalence of depressive symptoms in heart failure patients. One might expect fewer depressed patients to wish to participate in such studies. Further, no studies have evaluated cognitive impairment or depression specifically in the end stages of the condition, which is when physicians would be assessing patients' competence for PAS. If these are the results from patients in the community and patients prior to discharge from hospital, it would be reasonable to hypothesise that the results in the end stages would be much starker.

If assisted suicide were an available option there might be pressure for all severely ill people to consider it, even if they would not otherwise entertain such an idea. Feelings of being a burden on friends, family and the NHS may also come into play (House of Lords 2005, Mak *et al.* 2003, Savage 2002). Sceptics argue that this has the potential to lead to an avalanche of assisted deaths. In itself this might cut costs to the NHS as heart failure is a financial huge burden (Cowie & Zaphinou 2002, Taylor & Stott 2002). On the other hand, it could be argued that if the safeguards were stringent enough, PAS for heart failure patients would not be a cheap option for the NHS. There would need to be the option of an alternative, palliative care pathway and the provision of psychiatric physicians to cater for all our heart failure patients requesting PAS (Gibbs 1998).

The Church of England robustly rejects the idea of legalisation of voluntary assisted dying, suggesting that there is almost no reason for patients with an incurable condition to die in agony or distress with the developments in palliative care. Many agree with them (House of Lords 2005, Campbell 2002, Dunstan & Royal 1996, Savage 2002). However there are studies which suggest that intractable suffering does exist even with the intervention of palliative care (Kaldjian *et al.* 2004, Guedj *et al.* 2005, The SUPPORT principle investigators 1995).

Another interesting question which could be asked is this. Is there a difference in assisted dying and 'extreme' palliative care? The 'Doctrine of Double Effect' has traditionally permitted the use of high doses of strong and dangerous drugs in the palliative care of patients even where this puts the life of the patient at serious risk. This has been referred to as 'underground assisted dying' (Ward & Tate 1994, Kemp 2002, Shaw 2002, Magnusson 2004). Withholding or withdrawing life-prolonging treatment may be seen as morally equivalent to assisted dying (Doyal & Doyal 2001). It could be argued that the only difference here is the way in which the health-care professional construes the situation to make it feel morally correct. The distinction between killing and letting die is not a clear one and it has been argued that consequences which are intended and those that are foreseen but unintended is a distinction without a difference (House of Lords 2005).

The thought processes and reasons behind patients' requesting assisted death have been held to be similar to those thought processes of patients refusing life sustaining treatment (House of Lords 2005). Physicians are legally required to explain the consequences if we are to withdraw or withhold treatment by the request of that patient (Biggs 2001, Otlowski 2000). However when it is a physician's decision to withdraw life-prolonging treatment or initiate palliative care this is rarely discussed. Patients are given prescribed morphine when required and other concoctions to make them comfortable without the explanation that it may have the effect of shortening the duration of life. Shaw (2002) argues that there is little moral difference between direct and indirect killing. The author would argue that which ever way our patients die now or in the future, explanation and, where applicable, consent should surely be required. The consent process, after all, exists to protect patient autonomy and prevent harm (Beigler 2003, Shaw 2002).

So to conclude, what has become evident from the above debate is that if the legalisation of PAS ever occurs it may not be applicable for the heart failure population. Research into every aspect of end of life care is scant. Evidence for unmet needs in terminal heart failure has grown; however investigations into how to rectify the situation remain rudimentary. Extensive research needs to be directed into compiling prognostic models and guidelines for the heart failure patient's end of life. Research into depression and cognitive dysfunction is inconclusive and would need much more attention before we could safely consider heart failure patients for PAS. The bill as it stands is subjective, which may leave all patients with malignant and non-malignant diseases vulnerable to abuse.

At an empirical level, the existence of 'underground assisted dying' is difficult to deny in the form of voluntary and involuntary passive assisted dying. Currently pragmatics, not ethics, govern practice around assisted dying. PAS if legalised may never be perfectly safe but what is important is harm minimisation and acting in the best interests of our patients. However we first need to question the ethics behind practices that already exist. Perhaps arguments about assisted dying should concentrate on how best to regulate underground assisted dying, rather than introducing novel legislation to deal with poorly definable situations which may arbitrarily leave the heart failure patient behind.

Linda Gladman

References

Acanfora, D., Trojano, L., Iannuzzi, G.L., Furgi, G., Picone, C., Rengo, C., Abete, P. & Rengo, F. (1996). The brain in congestive heart failure. *Archives of Gerontology and Geriatrics*, 23, 247–56.

Allmark, P. (2002). Death with dignity. *Journal of Medical Ethics*, 28, 255–7.

Almeida, O. & Flicker, L. (2001). The mind of a failing heart: systematic review of the association between congestive heart failure and cognitive functioning. *International Medical Journal*, 31 (5), 290–301.

Anderson, H., Ward, C., Eardley, A., Gomm, S.A., Connolly, M., Coppinger, T., Corgie, D., Williams, J.L. & Makin, W.P. (2001). The concerns of patients under palliative care and a heart failure clinic are not being met. *Palliative Care Medicine*, 15, 279–86.

Antonelli, R *et al* (2003) Verbal memory impairment in congestive heart failure. *Journal of Clinical Neurophysiology*, 25 (1), 14–23.

Artinian, N.T., Artinian, C.G. & Saunders, M.M. (2004). Identifying and treating depression in patients with heart failure. *Journal of Cardiovascular Nursing*, 19 (65), 547–56.

Bennett, S. & Sauve, M. (2003). Cognitive deficits in patients with heart failure: A review of the literature. *The Journal of Cardiovascular Nursing*, 18 (3), 219–24.

Biegler, P. (2003). Should patients consent be required to write do not resuscitation orders. *Journal of Medical Ethics*, 29, 359–63.

Biggs, H. (2001). *Assisted dying. Death with Dignity and the Law*. Great Britain: Hart Publishing.

Cacciatore, F. (1998). Congestive heart failure and cognitive impairment in older population. *Journal of American Geriatric Society*, 46, 1343–8.

Campbell, L. (2002). On Dying Well: An Anglican contribution to the debate on assisted dying. *Journal of Medical Ethics*, 28, 209–10.

Cowie, M. & Zaphinou, A. (2002). Management of chronic heart failure. *British Medical Journal*, 325, 422–5.

Cushen, M. (1994). Palliative care in severe heart failure. *British Medical Journal*, 308, 717–18.

Davidson, P. M. (2002). Intergrated, collaborative palliative care in heart failure: The St. George Heart Service experience. *Journal of Cardiovascular Nursing*, 19 (1), 68–76.

Davies, S. (2002). Legalising active assisted dying and physician assisted suicide. *British Medical Journal*, 324, 846.

Department of Health (2002). *National Service Framework: Developing Services for Heart Failure*. www.dh.gov.uk 7/12/05.

Doyal, L. & Doyal, L. (2001). Why assisted dying and physician assisted suicide should be legalised. *British Medical Journal*, 323, 1079–80.

Dunstan, G. R. and Royal, P. J. L. (1996) Assisted dying: death, dying and the medical duty. *British Medical Journal*, 313, 1495–9.

Ekman, I. Fagerberg, B. & Skoog, I. (2001). The clinical implications of cognitive impairment in elderly patients with chronic heart failure. *Journal of Cardiovascular Nursing*, 16 (1), 47–9.

Ellershaw, J. & Ward, C. (2003). Care of the dying patient: the last hours of life. *British Medical Journal*, 326, 30–4.

Emanuel, E.J., Daniels, E.R., Fairclough, D.L. & Clarridge, B.R. (1998). The practice of euthanasia and physician-assisted suicide in the United States: adherence to proposed safeguards and effects on physicians. *Journal of American Medical Association*, 280, 507–13.

Frey, R.G. (2005) Pain, vivisection, and the value of life. *Journal of Medical Ethics*, 31, 202–4.

Friedman, M.M. & Griffin, J.A. (2001). Relationship of physical symptoms and physical functioning to depression in patients with heart failure. *Heart and Lung*, 30 (2), 98–104.

Garrard, E. & Wilkinson, S. (2005). Passive assisted dying. *Journal of Medical Ethics*, 31, 64–8.

Gibbs, M.L. (1998). Dying from heart failure lessons from palliative care. *British Medical Journal*, 317, 961–2.

Goodlin, S.J., Hauptman, P.J., Arnold, R., Grady, K., Hershberger, R.E., Kutner, J., Masoudi, F., Spertus, J., Dracup, K., Cleary, J.F., Medak, R., Crispell, K., Pina, I., Stuart, B., Whitney, C., Rector, T., Teno, J. & Renlund, D.G. (2004). Consensus statement palliative and supportive care in advanced heart failure. *Journal of Cardiac Failure*, 10 (3), 200–9.

Gottlieb, S.S., Khatta, M., Friedmann, E., Einbinder, L., Katzen, S., Baker, B., Marshall, J., Minshall, S, Robinson, S., Fisher, M.L., Potenza, M., Sigler, B., Baldwin, C. & Thomas, S.A. (2004). The influence of age, gender and race on the prevalence of depression in heart failure patients. *Journal of the American College of Cardiology*, 43 (9), 1542–9.

Guck, T.P., Elsasser, G.N., Kavan, M.G. & Barone, E.J. (2003). Depression and congestive heart failure. *Congestive Heart Failure*, 9 (3), 166–9.

Guedj, M.J., Gilbert, M., Maudet, A., Munoz Sastre, M.T., Mullet, E. & Sorum, P.C. (2005). The acceptability of ending a patient's life. *Journal of Medical Ethics*, 31, 311–17.

Hanratty, B., Hibbert, D., Mair, F., May, C., Ward, C., Capewell, S., Litva, A. & Corcoran, G. (2002). Doctors' perceptions of palliative care for heart failure: focus group study. *British Medical Journal*, 325, 581–5.

Havranek, E. P., Ware, M.G. & Lowes, B.D. (1999). Prevalence of depression in congestive cardiac failure. *American Journal of Cardiology*, 84, 348–50.

House of Lords (2005). *Assisted Dying for the Terminally Ill Bill*. London: The Stationery Office.

Jacob, S. & Sebastian, J. (2003). Depression and congestion heart failure: are anti-depressants underutilised? *European Journal of Heart Failure*, 5, 399–400.

Jones, S. (1995). Palliative care in terminal cardiac care. *British Medical Journal*, 310, 805–10.

Kaldjian, L.C., Jekel, J.F., Bernene, J.L., Rosenthal, G.E., Vaughan-Sarrazin, M. & Duffy, T.P. (2004). Internists attitudes towards terminal sedation in end of life care. *Journal of Medical Ethics*, 30, 499–503.

Kemp, N.D.A. (2002). Angels of death: Exploring the assisted dying underground. *British Medical Journal*, 325, 396–7.

Krumholz, H.M., Phillips, R.S., Hamel, M.B., Teno, J.M., Bellamy, P. Broste, S.K., Califf, R.M., Vidaillet, H., Davis, R.B., Mulbaier, L.H., Connors, A.F. jr.,Lynn, J. & Goldman, L. (1998). Resuscitation preferences among patients with severe congestive heart failure: results from SUPPORT project. Study to understand prognoses and preferences for outcomes and risks of treatments. *Circulation*, 98, 648–55.

Mak, Y.W., Elwyn, G. & Finlay, I.G. (2003). Patient's voices are needed in debate on assisted dying. *British Medical Journal*, 327, 213–15.

Magnusson, R.S. (2004. Assisted dying: above ground, below ground. *Journal of Medical Ethics*, 30, 441–6.

Mental Capacity Act (2005). Office of public sector information http://www.opsi.gov.uk 10/12/05.

Miller, A.B. (2002). Heart failure and depression. *European Journal of Heart Failure*, 4 (4), 401–2.

Assisted dying and heart failure

National Institute for Clinical Excellence (NICE) (2003). *Chronic heart failure. Management of chronic heart failure in adults in primary and secondary care.* www.nice.org.uk 7/12/05.

O'Brien, T., Welsh, J. & Dunn, F.G. (1998). ABC of palliative care: non-malignant conditions. *British Medical Journal*, **316**, 286–9.

Otlowski, M. (2000). *Voluntary assisted dying and the common law.* Oxford: Oxford University Press.

Onwuteaka-Philipsen, B.D., van der Heide, A., Muller, M.T., Rurup, M., Rietjens, J.A., Georges, J.J., Vrakking, A.M., Cuperus-Bosma, J.M., van der Wal, G. & van der Maas, P.J. (2005). Dutch experience of monitoring euthanasia. *British Medical Journal*, **331**, 691–3.

Riegel, B., Bennett, J.A., Davis, A., Carlson, B., Montague, J., Robin, H. & Glaser, D. (2002). Cognitive impairment in heart failure: issues of measurement and aetiology. *The Journal of Cardiovascular Nursing*, **11** (6), 520–9.

Rivett, A.G. (2002). Legalising active Assisted dying and physician assisted suicide. *British Medical Journal*, **324**, 846–56.

Rogers, A.E., Addington-Hall, J.M., Abery, A.J., McCoy, A.S., Bulpitt, C., Coats, A.J. & Gibbs, J.S. (2000). Knowledge and communication difficulties for patients with chronic heart failure: qualitative study. *British Medical Journal*. **321**, 605–7.

Rumsfeld, J. S. *et al.* (2003). Cardiovascular outcomes research consortium. *Journal of the American College of Cardiology*, **42** (10), 1811–17.

Savage, M. (2002). Legalising active assisted dying and physician assisted suicide: people's autonomy is not absolute. *British Medical Journal*, **324**, 846–56.

Shaw, A.B. (2002). Two challenges to the double effect doctrine: assisted dying and abortion. *Journal of Medical Ethics*, **28**, 102–4.

Sheldon, T. (2004). The good assisted dying Guide 2004: where, what, and who in choices in dying. *British Medical Journal*, **329**, 745–7.

Skotzko, C.E., Krichten, C., Zietowski, G., Alves, L., Freudenberger, R., Robinson, S., Fisher, M. & Gottlieb, S.S. (2000). Depression is common and precludes accurate assessment of functional status in elderly patients with congestive heart failure. *Journal of Cardiac Failure*, **6**, 300–5.

Sloan, R.H. (2002). Cancer isn't the only malignant disease. *British Medical Journal*, **324**, 1035–40.

Stainiforth, A.D., Kinnear, W.J. & Cowley, A.J. (2001). Cognitive impairment in heart failure with Cheyne-Stokes respiration. *Heart*, **85** (18), 18–22.

Taylor, J. & Stott, D.J. (2002). Chronic heart failure and cognitive impairment: co-existence of conditions or true association? *European Journal of Heart Failure*, **4** (1), 7–9.

The, A.M., Hak, T., Koeter, G. & van Der Wal, G. (2000). Collusion in doctor-patient communication about imminent death: an ethnographic study. *British Medical Journal*, **321**, 1376–81.

The SUPPORT principle investigators (1995). A controlled trial to improve care for the seriously ill hospitalised patients. The study to understand prognoses and preferences for outcomes and risks of treatments. *Journal of American Medical Association*, **274** (20), 1591–8.

Turvey, C.L., Schultz, K., Arndt, S., Wallace, R.B. & Herzog, R. (2002). Prevalence and correlates of depressive symptoms in a community sample of people suffering from heart failure. *Journal of Geriatric Society*, **50** (12), 2003–8.

Vaccarino, V. (2001). Depressive symptoms and risk of functional decline and death in patients with heart failure. *Journal of the American College of Cardiology*, **38** (1), 199–205.

Wal, G.V.D. & Dillmann, R.J. (1994). Assisted dying in the Netherlands. *British Medical Journal*, **308**, 1346–9.

Ward, B.J. & Tate P.A. (1994). Attitudes among NHS physicians to request for assisted dying. *British Medical Journal*, **308**, 1332–4.

Ward, C. (2002). The need for palliative care in the management of heart failure. *Heart*, **87** (3), 294–9.

Wehby, D. & Brenner, P. (1997). Perceived learning needs of patients with heart failure. *Heart Lung*, **28**, 21–40.

Wilson, K.G., Scott, J.F., Graham, I.D., Kozack, J.F., Chater, S., Viola, R.A., de Faye, B.J., Weaver, L.A. & Curran, D. (2000). Attitudes of terminally ill patients towards assisted dying and physician assisted suicide. *Archives of Internal Medicine*, **160**, 2454–60.

Zuccala, G. Onder, G. Pedone, C., Carosella, L., Pahor, M. & Bernabei, R. (2001). Hypotension and cognitive impairment: selective association in patients with heart failure. *Neurology*, **57** (11), 1986–92.

Zuccala, G . Cattel, C., Manes-Gravina, E., Di Niro, M.G., Cocchi, A. & Bernbei, R. (1997). Left ventricular dysfunction: a clue to cognitive impairment in older patients with heart failure. *Journal of Neurology Neurosurgery and Psychiatry*. **63** (4), 509–12.

Bibliography

Davis, R.C. & Hobbs, F.D.R. (2000). ABC of heart failure: history and epidemiology. *British Medical Journal*, 320, 39–42.

Glickman, M. (1998). Making palliative care better. *British Medical Journal,* 316, 319.

Moulder, E. (2002). Cancer isn't the only malignant disease. *British Medical Journal*, 324, 307–8.

Nordgren, L. & Olsson, H. (2003). Palliative care in a coronary care unit; a qualitative study of physicians and nurses perceptions. *Journal of Clinical Nursing*, 13, 185–93.

Stewart, S. (2002). Palliative care for heart failure. *British Medical Journal*, 325, 915–16.

Sullivan, M.D., Rapp, S., Fitzgibbon, D. & Chapman, C.R. (1997). Pain and the choice to hasten ones death in patients with painful metastic cancer. *Journal of Palliative Care*, 13 (3), 18–28.

New York Heart Association Scale

Appendix

New York Heart Association Scale (NYHA)

NYHA I Patients have no limitation on activities;
they suffer no symptoms from ordinary activities,
however there is evidence of left ventricular
impairment on echocardiography.

NYHA II Patients suffer with mild limitation of activity;
they are comfortable with rest or with mild exertion.
Evidence of mild to moderate left ventricular
impairment on echocardiography.

NYHA III Patients suffer marked limitation of activity;
they are comfortable only at rest.
Evidence of moderate to severe left ventricular
impairment on echocardiography

NYHA IV Patients confined to bed or chair;
even minimal activity brings on discomfort and
symptoms occur at rest. Evidence of severe left
ventricular impairment on echocardiography.

Index